LET'S TALK SH!T

DISEASE, DIGESTION, GUT HEALTH, AND FECAL TRANSPLANTS

SABINE HAZAN, MD

SHELI ELLSWORTH

THOMAS BORODY, MD

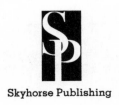

Skyhorse Publishing

Copyright © 2020, 2024 by Sabine Hazan, MD

All rights reserved. No part of this book may be reproduced in any manner without the express written consent of the publisher, except in the case of brief excerpts in critical reviews or articles. All inquiries should be addressed to Skyhorse Publishing, 307 West 36th Street, 11th Floor, New York, NY 10018.

Skyhorse Publishing books may be purchased in bulk at special discounts for sales promotion, corporate gifts, fund-raising, or educational purposes. Special editions can also be created to specifications. For details, contact the Special Sales Department, Skyhorse Publishing, 307 West 36th Street, 11th Floor, New York, NY 10018 or info@skyhorsepublishing.com.

Skyhorse® and Skyhorse Publishing® are registered trademarks of Skyhorse Publishing, Inc.®, a Delaware corporation.

Visit our website at www.skyhorsepublishing.com.

10 9 8 7 6 5 4 3 2 1

Library of Congress Control Number: 2024931405.

Cover design by Kai Texel
Cover artwork by Getty Images

ISBN: 978-1-5107-8081-1
Ebook ISBN: 978-1-5107-8131-3

Printed in the United States of America

This book was previously published as
Let's Talk Sh!t (ISBN: 9780578684703).

CONTENTS

FROM THE AUTHORS

Dr. Sabine Hazan has been a practicing gastroenterologist and clinical trial researcher for many years. Unafraid to get her hands dirty, Dr. Hazan has examined, studied, and observed a lot of excrement. When she asked me to help her with this book, I said that I would be honored to help her get her sh!t together. And although my voice became part of our writing collaboration, we use the pronoun "I" and its possessive forms to narrate from her point of view. —Sheli Ellsworth

Dr. Thomas Borody, our content editor, researcher, and my mentor is among the first clinicians who opened our minds and allowed us to step out of the box of conventional treatment methods. His editorial made this book a possibility and a gift to those who want to understand the possibilities of Fecal Microbiota Transplantation (FMT). —Sabine Hazan, M.D.

CHAPTER 1

BELLY ACHES

"All disease begins in the gut."
—Hippocrates

As a gastroenterologist for more than twenty-five years, most of the complaints I hear are related to bloating and weight gain. Some say they feel like they're six-months pregnant, others say everything they eat gives them gas. Then there's the middle-age mantra, "I don't overeat, but my waistline continues to grow." Some of us are gassy, some of us need to shed a few pounds, and—for some—our bowel movements are no more predictable than squirrels on the road. When it comes to our girth, few of us are 100 percent satisfied.

How much of our waistline woes are a result of what we eat? How much of it is under our control?

It would be irresponsible for me or anyone else to say that everyone's problem could be solved with one solution.

If it were possible that a particular diet would cure

> The **gut** is the segment of the gastrointestinal tract extending from the pyloric sphincter of the stomach to the anus.

everything from Crohn's disease to obesity, someone would have trade-marked it long ago. Whether you are a constipated comedienne, a flatulent flight attendant, or a portly postman, chances are your problems originate in your gastrointestinal (GI) tract. And it's not just digestive discomforts that start in your gut. From autism to zinc deficiencies, research is linking the viruses, bacteria, and fungi that colonize our GI tract to numerous disorders and to our overall health. These viruses, bacteria, and fungi are microorganisms (tiny forms of life that are too small to be seen by the naked eye) that make up what is known as the *intestinal biome*—a world of interdependent microbial communities located in the gut—mostly in the large intestine. And when you consider that these microorganisms process about thirty-five tons of food in our lifetime, they do work their tails off.

Originally, **C. diff** was classified as *Clostridium difficile*. In 2016, it was reclassified. *Clostridioides difficile (C. diff)* is a bacterium that causes diarrhea and inflammation of the colon. *C. diff* infections usually follow antibiotic use.

One in eleven people over age sixty-five die of a health-care-associated *C. diff* infection.

I have come to believe that these populations of microorganisms are the superheroes of our health. I have seen them cure life-threatening bacterial infections like *Clostridioides difficile* and I'm observing changes in obesity, heart disease, inflammatory bowel disease (IBD), as well as improvement in autism and psoriasis by the introduction of richer (more diverse) microbes. But why is gut health so important to overall health? This comes down to what happens in our intestinal biome and an understanding of how our bodies process food. How does this digestive distillation happen? And why do things go so wrong? First, we have to go over some basic sh!t.

CHAPTER 2

BIOME BASICS

"We depend on a vast army of microbes to stay alive:
a microbiome that protects us against germs, breaks down food to
release energy, and produces vitamins."
—Oxford Dictionary

The genes that compose our twenty-three chromosomes change over generations. This means that if a small genetic change (mutation) occurs, it will only enter the gene pool when we have children who carry these changes in their DNA. This slow transformation is good because it prevents us from bearing offspring who look like Teletubbies. However, our microbiome is far more dynamic.

Because bacterial generations are measured in hours not years, bacteria can adapt to change much faster than our own DNA. The flexibility of our microbiota allows us to adapt. If our diet changes, our microbiota compensate much faster than our DNA or our behavior. Ever try to feed beets to a three-year-old? Our gut bacteria will cooperate way before our toddler gets that hungry.

Microbes live in almost all environments: from high on Mt. Everest to deep in the Pacific Ocean's Mariana Trench. They live in the north and south poles, deserts, geysers, rocks, and volcanoes. Most of them are single-cell organisms or colonies of single-cell organisms that not only survive but can thrive in environments that otherwise appear inhospitable. Bacteria and viruses are unimaginably tiny and are usually measured in microns, which is abbreviated "µm." One micron equals one/one-millionth of a meter or about 0.00004 inches. Depending on the microbe, a couple of hundred thousand could sit on the head of a pin.

Our microbiome is all of the bacteria, viruses, and fungi that inhabit the human body. They are everywhere: skin, mouth, throat, stomach, colon, uterus, ovarian follicles, prostate, lungs, ears, and eyes. You name it and there are microorganisms nearby. About ten thousand different microbial species were identified by the Human Microbiome Project by 2014.

Microbiologists (those who study this vast world) divide bacteria into two categories: **aerobic**, meaning they require oxygen, and **anaerobic**, meaning they don't require oxygen. Bacteria that live on the skin are aerobic while those that thrive in the gut are usually anaerobic.

Joshua Lederberg (1925–2008) coined the term microbiome "to signify the ecological community of commensal, symbiotic, and pathogenic micro-organisms that literally share our body space" (Lederberg and McCray 2001). Lederberg, at the age of thirty-three won the 1958 Nobel Prize in Physiology or Medicine for essentially discovering that bacteria are capable of mating and exchanging genes.

THE GOOD

Microbes perform functions that our bodies could otherwise never manage. Not only do they turn food into energy (through fermentation and sulphate reduction of carbohydrates), but their population numbers adapt to our lifestyle. And yes, they are moving, eating, sleeping, and reproducing just like any life form—enough to make us want to swallow an antihistamine and take a hot steamy shower. In fact, these little critters outnumber human tissue cells ten to one and make up about five pounds of our total weight.

TYPES OF ANAEROBES:
Obligate anaerobes are harmed by oxygen.
Aerotolerant anaerobes cannot use oxygen for growth but tolerate its presence.
Facultative anaerobes grow without oxygen but use oxygen if it is present.

Our microbes are as much a part of our bodies as tattoos and much more practical, unless you happen to have a tattoo of the New York City subway system. They are our biological family, and we are theirs. *We only exist because they exist.* It is a completely interdependent relationship. Our microbiome is an organ system that is as critical for our survival as our brain or our heart.

It's in the intestines where most microbiota influence our immune system, and where many of our body's metabolic processes are conceived. Vitamins like B12 are produced by lactic acid bacteria. *Bifidobacteria* makes folate. Other vitamins synthesized by gut bacteria include vitamin K, pantothenic acid, thiamine, riboflavin, biotin, and more. It is also where toxins are broken down and invading bacteria are euthanized. It's here, where the magic happens, in which I specialize.

SCIENTIFIC CLASSIFICATIONS OF BACTERIA:
Commensal bacteria benefit where other bacteria neither benefit nor are harmed.
Mutualistic bacteria benefit from each other.
Parasitic bacteria benefit at the expense of the host.
Pathogenic bacteria are known to cause disease (see p. 15).

It is also where bacteria like *E. coli* (*Escherichia coli*) and *Salmonella* (widely known to cause food poisoning) live and are normally kept in check by their more well-behaved bacterial counterparts. This brings up another important concept: location, location, location.

Another example, *H. pylori* (*Helicobacter pylori*) is a bacterium that protects against cancer of the esophagus. However, the exact same strain can cause ulcers and even stomach cancer. Where bacteria practice their craft and their ratios to other bacteria determine their functional relevance (goodness or badness). So, instead of good and bad, I tend to think of them as pious (usually good) or agnostic (neither good nor bad). Science uses terms like mutualist, commensal, pathogenic, and parasitic. See page 8.

> **PIOUS BACTERIA:**
> - *Actinobacteria*
> - *Bacteroidetes*
> - *Bifidobacterium*
> - *Firmicutes*
> - *Lachnospiraceae*
> - *Lactobacillus*
> - *Prevotellaceae*
> - *Proteobacteria*
> - *Rikenellaceae*
> - *Streptococcus thermophilus*

The bacterium, *Akkermansia muciniphila* is thought to colonize in the mucus layer of the colon, as well as maintaining and strengthening the gut barrier. Several metabolic processes profit from its existence. It has been postulated to alleviate inflammation and reduce weight gain when fed to mice (Zhao et al., 2017). However, in abundance, it can be associated with colon cancer. We don't know why or what the link is, but it would be difficult to classify *A. muciniphila* as good or bad until we do further tests and understand all these microbes in their environment.

THE BAD?

Traditional Western medicine is based on the doctrines of French chemist Louis Pasteur (1822–1895). Pasteur's main theory is known as the Germ Theory of Disease. Pasteur believed that microbes from an external source invaded the body and caused infectious disease. The concept of specific bacteria causing specific diseases became officially accepted as the foundation of Western medicine and microbiology in the late nineteenth century. Find the bad bug, kill the bad bug, all is well. Antibiotics were a natural outcropping from Pasteur's theory.

Pierre Jacques Antoine Béchamp (1816–1908) was another French scientist known for his breakthroughs in organic chemistry and for his bitter rivalry with Louis Pasteur. Béchamp claimed that unfavorable hosts and environmental conditions disrupted native microzymas (Béchamp's name for the "molecular granulations" in biological fluids that were the elementary units of life) whereupon they decomposed host tissue by producing pathogenic bacteria. His disagreement with Pasteur led to efforts to have his work placed on the *Index Librorum Prohibitorum* (books prohibited by the Catholic Church). A brief obituary, in the *British Medical Journal* when Béchamp died, noted that Béchamp was "associated with bygone controversies as to priority which it would be unprofitable to recall" (Manchester, 2007).

Béchamp was wrong, but not completely wrong.

AGNOSTIC BACTERIA:

- *Bacillus cereus*
- *Campylobacter*
- *Candida albicans*
- *Clostridium difficile*
- *Helicobacter pylori*
- *Listeria*
- *Salmonella*
- *Shigella*
- Shiga toxin-prod. *E. coli*
- *Yersinia*

His idea that microorganisms are imperative to health, and the idea that microbiota are only pathogenic under the wrong conditions, or in the wrong place, is now accepted by researchers who study the microbiology of animals and plants.

So, while bacteria themselves are neither good nor bad, a bacteria's usefulness (fitness) is dependent on how it interacts with the genetics of its host (human), the microorganisms it interacts with (microbiome), and environmental factors like diet, chemicals, and antibiotics (Ehrlich, Hiller, & Hu, 2008). Additionally, because a single species will have a variety of strains, we can't simply look at a particular species and label it pathogenic. Even *E. coli* has a variety of strains. Most of our *E. coli* cliques do important digestive work by helping us absorb iron (Han & Qi, 2018). But while some *E. coli* are very helpful and aid in digestion, others are just plain infectious and can leave us worshipping the porcelain throne with a urinary tract infection or a life-affirming case of vomiting and diarrhea. Hence, we recognize that some species are more commonly commensal while others are more commonly pathogenic—often a host-related behavior.

Some bacteria have the ability to behave well for long periods of time. For example, *Pneumococcus* bacteria live in our nose and the back of our mouth usually without causing trouble. Then our immune system tanks for whatever reason (age, illness, environmental stressors) and *Pneumococcus* can cause pneumonia.

Many bacteria have the ability to remain in a persistent dormant state if they are forced to by environmental factors like antibiotic treatment (Venkova, Yeo, & Espinosa, 2018). *Mycobacterium tuberculosis* is the bacterium that causes tuberculosis. It can lay dormant or latent for long periods of time, making it extremely resistant to the immune system and drug treatment. Researchers at the University of Copenhagen (2018) studied *E. coli* from patients with urinary tract infections supposedly under control with antibiotic treatment. In time, the bacteria re-awoke and began to re-infect.

Occasionally, we get an influx of street-gang bacteria or a biome shift that will allow what some might call "pathogenic" bacterium to multiply. These outbreaks are often called infections and may cause fever, vomiting, and diarrhea, etc.

Tetanus, typhoid fever, diphtheria, and syphilis are examples of infections by bacteria usually considered pathogenic. However, some people carry the bacteria *Salmonella typhi* and have no obvious symptoms of illness. They are considered asymptomatic carriers, which is another reason why classification of bacteria as good and bad can be so challenging.

But fortunately, only a small percentage of our body's bacteria have been identified as disease-causing (pathogenic).

A study by Furuya-Kanamori, et al. (2015) found *Clostridium difficile* or *C. diff* to be the most common hospital infection. However, it is also found in 18–90 percent of newborns, up to 15 percent in the general population, and up to 51 percent in the elderly living in care facilities with no symptoms of illness. However, our company, Progenabiome, found that out of one thousand patients, 100 percent had non toxigenic *C. diff* imprint in their stools. This may indicate that *C. diff* is not transmitted from person to person by hand transmission or from hospital workers but becomes toxic when bacterial diversity is decreased. In a natural environment,

RISK FACTORS FOR *C. DIFF*:

- Being sixty-five or older
- Recent hospitalization
- Weakened immune system
- Previous *C. diff* infection
- Antibiotic therapy
- Non-surgical gastrointestinal procedures
- Presence of a nasogastric tube
- Anti-ulcer therapy

the species of living organisms keep each other in check. Same goes in the gut, the more you kill off the diverse bacteria, the more imbalance you have and thus disease.

In 2005, the mortality rate for *C. diff* toxin hospitalizations was 9.7 percent. So, while 10 percent of infected hospitalized people die from this bacterium, many people have the bacterium in their microbiome and suffer no known symptoms because of its presence.

The overall low numbers of disease-causing microbes in most humans suggests that people acquire disease-causing microbes from outside environmental sources and our own bacterial sheriffs usually keep them in check.

This leads to the conclusion that most of our microbiome is beneficial and prevents illness. It is an imbalance of our microbiota (dysbiosis) that causes disease.

THE ALTERNATIVE

With all of this in mind, I want you to consider that we can no longer treat disease as simple eradication, committing microbial genocide with antibiotics. Think of wellness and disease as a complex interplay with us as the host and these microbes as our delightful but occasionally ill-behaved children. And, with the advent of genome sequencing technology (metagenomics), we are able to identify and count our children without resorting to different-colored monogrammed T-shirts.

The most comprehensive data about microbiome population numbers comes from the MetaHIT Consortium and Human Microbiome Project. Launched by the United States National Institutes of Health (NIH) in 2007, the Human Microbiome Project is research dedicated to understanding our microflora and its role in disease. The MetaHIT (Metagenomics of the Human Intestinal Tract) project is a European consortium of eight countries dedicated to understanding the microbiome and its relationship to inflammatory bowel disease and obesity.

This combined data identified more than ten thousand different species of microorganisms in the human GI tract. About four hundred of them are anaerobes (organisms that don't require oxygen) found only in the mouth and GI tract.

The microbiota populations in our bodies are as unique as fingerprints. The same research found that these populations vary by country, indicating that diet, genes, and environment all play a role in their development. A review of the research by Price, Abu-Ali, and Huttenhower in 2016 concluded that our individual microbiomes exhibit a high degree of bacterial diversity both within our bodies and between human subjects, making it difficult to define what a "healthy microbiome" encompasses.

The Human Microbiome Project discovered two opportunistic bacteria: *Staphylococcus aureus* and *Escherichia coli* in 15–30 percent of people tested. These bacteria, according to Broad Institute (2010), account for 36 percent of clinical infections requiring hospitalization.

We know that treating infection by repeated exposures to antibiotics has a tendency to decrease microbial richness (diversity), both in numbers and kind. But we also know that it can result in antibiotic-resistant strains of bacteria. Antibiotic-resistant *Staphylococcus aureus* and *Escherichia coli* strains have been observed worldwide and are a major concern in global public health. The future of treating infection may include using select bacteria harvested for a particular symbiotic function rather than simple eradication. This is possible by using next-generation genetic sequencing.

HOST GENES PLAY A PART

Research suggests that there is a relationship between certain human genes and some bacterial populations. Studies by Hsu et al. (2007) demonstrated that leptin deficient mice were more susceptible to infection by certain bacteria (*Streptococcus pneumoniae*). This means that genes indirectly (via leptin in this case) control how bacteria affect us.

Another example is tolerance for non-human produced milk as adults. Adults who lack the gene for digesting lactase but still consume milk are more likely to have abundant *Bifidobacteria* (Goodrich et al., 2017), which allows retailers to sell Chunky Monkey ice cream to people who would otherwise end up bloated and miserable.

> **Leptin** is a genetically driven hormone produced by fat cells that regulates appetite and tells us when we are full by sending signals to the hypothalamus in the brain.

The MyD88 gene is another gene thought to be linked to bacteria. Cani and Everard (2015) deleted this gene in a strain of mice. This gene is thought to be an important interface between microorganisms and host metabolism. When the mice were switched to a high fat diet, they were resistant to obesity, fat development, and insulin resistance. Their conclusion was that without the genes' relay to gut microbes, no additional weight could be gained.

Several types of arthritis are linked to the presence of the HLA-B27 gene which is known to promote an inflammatory response that starts in gut mucosa causing dysbiosis and spreading to the joints (Constantino et al., 2015).

> **Dysbiosis** is a disturbance or imbalance of our microbiota usually caused by the normally dominate species to be underrepresented and the normally contained species increasing to fill the void. Dysbiosis is most commonly diagnosed as small intestinal bacterial overgrowth (SIBO). More recently, dysbiosis is a term for an increase in the relative abundance of a certain group of bacteria which is thought to cause disease.

THE BEGINNING

How did this crazy, complex, co-dependent family get started? Without getting into the whole chicken-and-egg conundrum, it starts like all crazy co-dependent families—at birth. There is research that indicates we begin to acquire microbiota in the womb and birth canal (Perez-Muñoz, Arrieta, Ramer-Tait, & Walter, 2017). In fact, vaginally delivered infants verses Cesarean deliveries have higher num-

The term **Cesarean** was thought to be derived from the surgical birth of Julius Caesar, who later decreed that women endangered by childbirth must be cut open; hence, cesarean. Later, research revealed that an imperial law in Rome known as the *Lex Caesarea* was in effect from the time of Numa Pompilius (715-673 BC)— well before Caesar's time. The Latin word *caedere* means "to cut," which is also where the name Caesar came from.

bers of *Lactobacilli bacteria* during their first few days of life. *Lactobacilli* produce an acid that keeps potentially harmful opportunistic bacteria from colonizing.

As babies, we are exposed to our mother's bacteria in breastmilk. Then, before long we are toddling around putting every bacteria-laden thing imaginable in our mouths—keys, toys, shoes, dropped binkies, and the occasional bug. There is no shortage of ways to acquire bacteria, viruses, and fungi. They are in our foods, the air we breathe, and everything we touch. But once natural selection steps in, their numbers seek an equilibrium. By age two and a half, toddler microbiota begins to resemble that of an adult, although certain microbes thrive at different times in our developmental lives.

> **Natural selection** is the process where organisms better suited to their environment survive and produce more offspring, thereby passing their DNA on to the next generation. This applies to plants, animals, and microorganisms.

For example, in tweens, the gut microbiota is rich with organisms that encourage the production of vitamin B12 and folate, which promote growth. You remember that adolescent summer when you outgrew your clothes, or your shoe size ballooned to a point where your feet looked like they belonged to a clown. In adulthood, the intestinal microbiota ratio is usually more constant but dynamic enough to adapt to change.

However, diet also shapes our microbiota based on the amount of carbohydrates in our dietary fiber. Extreme animal or plant-based diets result in drastic differences in gut microbiota. In research done by De Filippo et al. (2010), African infants whose diets are dominated by starch and fiber harbor *Bacteroidetes* at 58 percent and *Actinobacteria* at 10 percent. Whereas, European children—whose diets are rich in sugar, starch, and animal protein—harbor only 22 percent Bacteroidetes and 7 percent *Actinobacteria*. Research suggests that our normal *Western* diet may even cause a microbial imbalance or dysbiosis because of a dearth of MAC (Microbiota-Accessible Carbohydrates: foods with roughage, like vegetables, fruits, and legumes).

Researchers think that some of our bacteria is much like our ancient bacterial archetypes, but that "human microbiomes have lost ancestral microbial diversity while becoming specialized for animal-based diets" (Moeller et al., 2014).

There is also reason to believe that there are distinct microbial communities made up of different clusters of bacteria. Researchers Arumugam et al. (2011) studied 1511 bacterial genomes of thirty-nine people from around the world and found three different bacterial population ratios (enterotypes). These types were not specific to nations or continents. However, some research has not supported the finding.

It is important to know that an abundance of one type of bacteria or another cannot characterize the functional complexity of our microbiome. Species that occur in lower numbers are sometimes the biggest producers. For example: *Escherichia*, low in abundance, contribute over 90 percent of two abundant proteins.

After our intestinal biomes become a more balanced or eubiotic population, events such as antibiotics, hygiene, smoking, depression, moving to a different environment, food pathogens, or even too many tequila shots at your cousin's wedding can cause one part of the family's population numbers to explode. This dysbiosis is at the root of many diseases.

As we age, some microbiota-dependent processes like our ability to produce short-chain fatty acids begin to wane. Others (like our ability to break down proteins) increase, which is a good reason to order that high protein plate off of the seniors' menu.

Before we get into the seedy back alley of my world, let's take it from the top.

No bad bugs! Even though we refer to some bacteria as bad or **pathogenic,** this is a label we usually ascribe when a bacterium has taken over more than its fair share of the environment and has become infectious. Even in a healthy microbiome, we find bacteria like *C. diff* but in smaller amounts.

CHAPTER 3

DIGESTIVE DISCOURSE

"Happiness is a good bank account,
a good cook, and good digestion."
—Jean-Jacques Rousseau

Is anyone's digestive tract normal? An ideal digestive anatomy and physiology does exist, although everyone suffers at some point with his/her digestion. However, there is a difference in "normal" suffering and those who suffer because of some sort of ailment or abnormality. Therefore, no one has a perfect gut. But there is an *anatomical norm* that most of us have.

The twisted path that leads to most digestive dilemmas, whether we are looking at something as severe as celiac disease or as treatable as flatulence, is about thirty feet long. Our gastrointestinal symphony starts at the mouth and finishes at the anus, with each part of the orchestra initiating a specific movement.

The whole digestive process is actually launched before you put food in your mouth. When you smell food, like fajitas at your favorite Mexican restaurant, a signal goes to your brain. One whiff causes those stale chips and salsa to taste soooo good! This stimulus also causes you to salivate (Dodds, Roland, Edgar, & Thornhill, 2015) and secrete acid in your stomach, both of which will ultimately help break down and digest those enchiladas and burritos that follow.

MOUTH

Our mouth is teeming with bacteria. Over six hundred different species of microbiota live there. Some of these bacteria (anaerobes) hide under the gumline and burrow deep in pockets of bone loss that form around teeth as a result of periodontal disease. Our saliva mostly contains benign strains of *Streptococcus* bacteria.

Researchers at the Max Planck Institute for Evolutionary Anthropology found that salivary bacteria ratios are as individual as we are. Geography, diet, or environment appears to have little effect on the kinds and numbers of bacteria found in saliva.

Research has also found certain types of salivary bacteria closely linked to tooth decay (Yang et al., 2014) and heart disease and (Nakano, Matsumoto, & Ooshima, 2010). Saliva testing is already used to diagnose some viral and bacterial infections.

Chew! Your mom probably told you to "Chew your food," while you were gobbling faster than Rosanne Barr and Megyn Kelly on their way out of network

Sore throats can be caused by bacteria or viruses like the cold virus. Bacterial infections like the streptococcus bacteria, a.k.a. **strep throat**, will sometimes have telltale white spots in the back of the throat. Strep can be confirmed with an in-office rapid strep test. Strep should be treated by a doctor since it can cause rheumatic fever and/or heart valve complications. Another cause of sore throat is **tonsillitis**. Tonsillitis can be caused by bacteria or viruses.

Additionally, researchers at the University of Manchester in the United Kingdom have found that chewing your food releases helper (Th17) cells, which are part of the immune system. These cells target harmful pathogens without impacting the beneficial bacteria in your body and mouth. Simply chewing your food, until it's soft, may assist in fighting inflammatory conditions of all kinds.

Despite the research, obsessive cud chewers like cattle are not rocket scientists, so don't count on chewing for IQ points.

television. Momma was right. The better you chew your food, the less work you give your stomach.

According to Ohio State University (Hollis & Zhu, 2014), chew softer foods five to ten times per mouthful and denser foods like meats and raw fruits and vegetables up to thirty times before swallowing. University of Pennsylvania suggests thirty to fifty times per mouthful for denser products. Food not broken down properly can cause bacterial overgrowth which leads to indigestion, bloating, and constipation.

Chewing also appears to lower circulating levels of ghrelin (Yagi, Ueda, Amitani, Asakawa, Miyawaki, & Inui, 2012), the hunger hormone, which is why chewing more is related to weighing less.

According to research by Allen and Smith (2015), chewing, even gum, is actually good for your brain because of the mouth's proximity to several key neural connections. Chen, Iinuma, Onozuka, and Kub (2015) found multiple neural circuits connecting the masticatory organs and the hippocampus. Both animal and human studies indicated that the brain is influenced by mastication. Unfortunately, some gum chewers swallow air which can result in gassiness.

ESOPHAGUS

Once food is chewed and swallowed, it transfers from the back of the mouth and down the esophagus, unless you were at a party, in which case your food might come back up anywhere—including your boss's designer sofa. (This brings up the most common problem in the esophagus: irritation caused by stomach acids.)

Occasionally, in immunosuppressed individuals, an overgrowth of fungi, yeast, or bacteria can also set off infectious esophagitis, causing swelling and irritation. Common symptoms of infectious esophagitis are pain and difficulty

> ## TYPES OF *ESOPHAGITIS:*
>
> - **Caustic.** Irritation from inhaling chemicals.
> - **Drug-induced**. Due to improper swallowing of un-coated medications.
> - **Eosinophilic**. Caused from food allergies.
> - **Infectious.** Can be due to a viral (Herpes simplex, Cytomegalovirus), fungal (Candida), parasitic, or bacterial infection.
> - **Lymphocytic.** Discovered in 2006. Noticeable increase in the amount of lymphocytes. This type is associated with Crohn's disease, reflux, and celiac disease.

when swallowing. And since over a hundred different types of microbes have been identified in the esophagus (Pei, Yang, Peek, Levine, Pride, & Blaser, 2005) a few of them may misbehave. Individuals receiving treatments like chemotherapy or medication for AIDS are especially vulnerable to esophageal infections.

There is even cause to believe there is a link between throat cancer and its resident bacteria (Chocolatewala, Chaturvedi, & Desale, 2010). Viruses can also wreak havoc in the mouth and throat. The sexually transmitted human papilloma virus (HPV) is responsible for a large percentage of oral and throat cancers (Kim, 2016). According to the CDC, HPV is thought to cause 70 percent of oropharyngeal cancers in the United States. Oral sex and deep kissing can be a method of HPV transmission. The likelihood of contracting oral HPV is directly associated with the number of sexual partners a person has had.

The esophagus eventually connects to the stomach via a muscular valve-like mechanism called the lower esophageal sphincter or LES junction. The LES should close after food goes though and stay closed for the stomach to do a thorough job.

LOWER ESOPHAGEAL SPHINCTER

If your diet is full of fried and fatty foods your LES may have a difficult time closing. This allows stomach acids to slosh back into the esophagus causing heartburn, also known as acid reflux. Those party foods like coffee, chocolate, mint, alcohol, and fat also weaken the valve, hindering the stomach's ability to process food— which is why my practice peaks in those post-holiday months. When this muscular valve relaxes too frequently (chronic), it is usually diagnosed as gastroesophageal reflux disease (GERD).

Many physicians find that the following lifestyle modifications or some over-the-counter meds can bring the irritating effects of infrequent heartburn to a complete halt.

If you have GERD, stop smoking. Tobacco can inhibit the production of saliva and may also relax the muscle between the esophagus and the stomach. Not good when you're trying to keep a meal down or impress a date.

Lose weight if you're out of shape. Decreasing abdominal pressure will make stomach acid leakage or backflow less likely in GERD sufferers.

Don't eat two to three hours before going to bed. If your body is horizontal, it's that much easier for your stomach acid to make its way

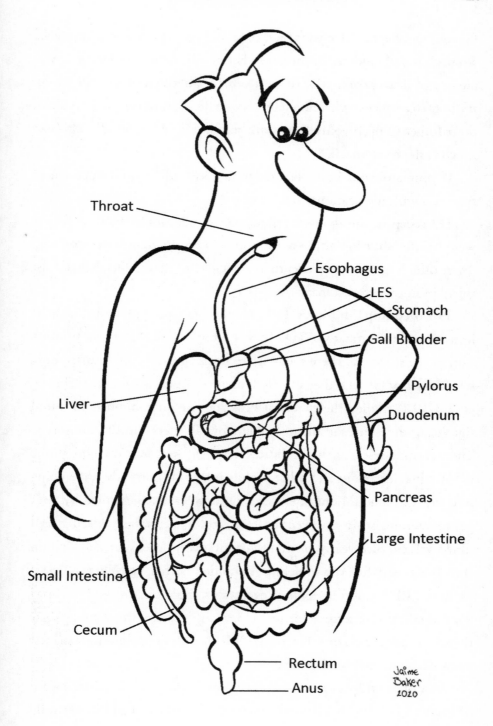

up your esophagus. Give your food time to digest so that the acid in your stomach is no longer being produced before you decide to snooze. If you are one of those people who sit to watch TV after a meal and fall asleep, try to take a quick walk beforehand, and when you return to your chair, don't forget to prop yourself up with pillows. It will make *The Bachelor* much easier to stomach.

If your problems have been diagnosed as GERD, your doctor may treat you with medications.

H2 receptor antagonists (which can sometimes be found OTC as well) help by shutting off 75 percent of acid production in the stomach. These offer longer-lasting relief than antacids but should be taken at least thirty minutes before a meal.

Proton pump inhibitors (PPIs) are another type of prescription medication used to combat GERD. They inhibit 90 percent of acid production in the stomach. These meds are recommended for those with more severe cases of GERD; they often eliminate symptoms altogether. Takagi et al. (2018) studied the effects of PPIs and the microbiome and found significant differences in the microbiota of PPI users and PPI non-users. There is some research that indicates that PPI users may be more prone to intestinal infections and other problems that are currently undergoing scrutiny. PPIs should only be used long term when prescribed by your gastroenterologist. In the event of long-term usage, patients need creatinine levels checked yearly, blood cell counts every other year, and vitamin B12 levels every five years (Nehra, Alexander, Loftus, & Nehra, 2018)

If GERD symptoms persist even after these treatments, you may require additional testing for an underlying medical condition. Since there is no simple diagnostic test for GERD, your physicians may suggest a few of the following diagnostic tools.

An **upper endoscopy** may be performed as a more accurate means of diagnosing GERD. Using this method, a doctor will administer mild sedation, then insert a small flexible tube with a camera on the end down your throat. The camera will enable the doctor to see if there are questionable or inflamed areas in the esophagus. In some cases, the doctor may pass small forceps or tissue scissors though the tube to perform a biopsy. Using tiny tweezers passed through the tube, the doctor can take a small sample of tissue from your esophagus to view through a microscope to see if it has been damaged because of stomach acid, infection, or other reasons.

Esophageal pH monitoring involves a small device that is inserted into the esophagus for twenty-four to forty-eight hours. This device stays with you throughout the day while you go about your business and monitors the amount of acid that enters your esophagus. This test provides doctors with an idea of how serious your heartburn might be.

STOMACH

The stomach is a muscular organ located in the left upper abdomen. The stomach secretes acid and enzymes so as to digest food. Ridges of muscle tissue called *rugae* line the stomach. Rugae unfold to accommodate a full stomach then contract, churning food to enhance digestion. Due to the high acidity of the stomach, most microorganisms cannot survive, but there are a few basic bacterial inhabitants of the stomach: *Streptococcus, Staphylococcus, Lactobacillus,* and *Peptostreptococcus.* These bacteria are usually present, but rarely at an infectious level.

However, one bacterium, *Helicobacter pylori* or **H. pylori** is a common stomach bacteria that can cause chronic gastritis (irritation of the stomach lining) and peptic ulcers

> **Antigens** are usually proteins on the surface of cells, viruses, fungi, or bacteria that stimulate our immune systems to produce antibodies.

(sores). *H. pylori* is also a carcinogen for gastric cancer. Symptoms of *H. pylori* infection include abdominal pain that worsens when your stomach is empty, nausea, loss of appetite, frequent burping, bloating, and weight loss.

A blood or stool **antigen test** can diagnose an *H. pylori* infection. *H. pylori* can also be diagnosed with a **urea breath test**. *H. pylori* is usually treated with antibiotics. Natural remedies like Manuka honey (made in Australia and New Zealand by bees that pollinate the native Manuka bush) have been known to keep *H. pylori* levels below the carcinogenic threshold, but more research is needed. Other natural remedies like lemon grass oil and certain probiotics are occasionally prescribed. More research is needed with natural products. All treatment should be followed up with testing.

Anyone who has seen the movie *In Cold Blood* knows that stomach ulcers and possibly psychopathic behavior may be the result of using nonsteroidal anti-inflammatory drugs (**NSAIDs** are aspirin, ibuprofen, and naproxen) like they are candy. These over-the-counter medicines can lower the blood's ability to clot, and specifically *aspirin* inhibits substances that protect the stomach lining.

When your digestive tract is operating normally, food should stay no longer than four hours in your stomach—even comfort food. After that, it can develop and produce gas.

> **Chyme** is what food becomes in the stomach. It is a thick fluid made of partially digested food and secretions that are formed during digestion.

A condition called **gastroparesis** occurs when your stomach takes too long to empty food. Gastroparesis sufferers may experience vomiting, nausea, bloating, pain, acid reflux, and fullness after only a few bites.

Your doctor may alter your diet and activities as well as prescribe medicines to improve gastric emptying.

In the stomach, acids produced while you were chewing start breaking food down into tiny particles small enough to go through another valve-like entrance called the *pylorus*.

PYLORUS

Pylorus means gatekeeper in Latin. Think of it as a spam filter for the small intestine. In order for food to enter the small intestine, food particles (chyme) need to be about half the thickness of a dime. Anything else gets bounced back. Occasionally, the pylorus will narrow causing pyloric stenosis. This condition is more common in infants (more so in male infants).

If you have abdominal swelling relieved only by vomiting or have forceful vomiting after eating, followed by hunger or dehydration, you may have a pyloric obstruction. Weight loss and contractions across the stomach after nursing or eating are common. Pyloric stenosis is usually treated surgically.

SMALL INTESTINE

Once food passes through the pylorus it enters the duodenum or first part of the small intestine. Here, bile from the gallbladder and digestive juices from the pancreas are mixed with the food. The small intestine is a folded or coiled tube as thick as the middle finger and about twenty to twenty-five feet long or about as wide as a tennis court. Food may loiter in the small intestine for up to two days, but because of acids and anti-microbials, bacterial growth is limited.

Ninety percent of our food is absorbed in the small intestine, which is why it's not in a hurry and travels only about six inches per hour or about the same speed as congress.

Research suggests that small-bowel microbes regulate both digestion and absorption of fats in the small intestine.

SIBO

Bloating, pain, and diarrhea can be a symptom of bacterial overgrowth—too many bacteria in the upper part of the small intestine. Symptoms occur immediately after eating because some bacteria come to the party early and begin to consume food in the small intestine and stay late before it can be absorbed. This is referred to as small intestinal bacterial overgrowth (SIBO).

These bacteria emit hydrogen and other gases which cause bloating and diarrhea.

SYMPTOMS OF SMALL INTESTINAL BACTERIAL OVERGROWTH (SIBO):

- Abdominal discomfort
- Bloating and distention
- Constipation
- Diarrhea
- Gas and belching

In more severe cases:

- Fatigue
- Weakness
- Weight loss
- Symptoms related to vitamin deficiencies

SIBO can be a result of abnormal motility in the small intestine and diminished gastric acid secretion. Disturbances in gut immune function and anatomical abnormalities of the GI tract also increase the likelihood of developing SIBO.

Our small intestine uses a series of muscle contractions to push food through. When the intestinal contractions don't move the bacteria out because the contractions are weak or disorganized, the bacteria grow out of control.

I like to think of the small bowel as a hose that is all twisted. If there is a blockage anywhere in the hose because of external compression or internal compression, food backs up and bacteria and pressure accumulate. Bacteria accumulates in areas where motion is not steady. Much like a clogged hose or pipe where crud accumulates. The compression can be secondary to an external compression from a tumor, fat process, scar tissues, endometrial tissue, enlarged organ or an anomaly. Internal blockage can be caused by a tumor.

Lastly, blockage and bacterial overgrowth can also be caused by damage to the nerves that stimulate the bowels, the connective tissue, or muscles that make up the small bowel. In essence, bacterial overgrowth is not just bacterial but usually secondary to something else preventing the bowel from moving regularly. When all etiologies are ruled out, all you're left with is dysbiosis.

IBS

For most, Cheerios travel through our intestines without our awareness. But for those with irritable bowel syndrome (IBS), these muscle contractions are associated with pain. While the cause of IBS is unknown, it's thought to be a result of abnormal gastrointestinal (GI) tract movements and a disruption in the communication between the brain and the GI tract. This abnormal motility of the small intestine is also associated with bloating, nausea, vomiting, and constipation. See page 52.

Other digestive problems that affect the small intestine include ulcers (uncommon), celiac disease, Crohn's disease, cancer (uncommon), and obstructions usually caused by scar tissue or hernias.

LARGE INTESTINE

After most nutrients are absorbed in the small intestine, the remaining fiber and waste move to the large intestine where water and salts are reabsorbed into your body. The large intestine, or the **Super Hero InTestine** (the **SH!T**), is also known as the colon. The colon is about five to six feet long and made of dense muscle tissue. Its divisions, in order from the small intestine down are the cecum, the ascending colon, the transverse colon, the descending colon, the sigmoid colon, the rectum, and the anal canal.

While previous parts of the digestive tract are fair to middlin' in microorganisms, the colon is flush, especially the **cecum**. The cecum is located in the lower right side of your abdomen. It is the widest part of your entire colon and is approximately five centimeters long, or a third as long as the average pen. The cecum gets the brunt of the small intestine's leftovers or food that escapes digestion. Here, the lining in a healthy human is at its thickest and crucial for the microbial environment. Microbes attach to the lush mucus lining and begin to break down those food molecules even further.

It is believed that the cecum contains one hundred times more bacteria than the small intestine. These bacteria are more diverse and anaerobes (like *Prevotellaceae*, *Lachnospiraceae*, and *Rikenellaceae*), which process those undigested complex carbohydrates. The cecum is also the storage of all bacteria, "the mother ship," if you will. It acts as a storage container as peristalsis in that location occurs backwards. The bowel

> **Microbiota-accessible carbohydrates** or MACs are undigestible carbohydrates from foods like bananas, beans, broccoli, cabbage, cauliflower, Brussels sprouts, and whole grains that are resistant to digestion in the small intestine, but in the large intestine are fermented or metabolized. MACs feed gut microbes by turning them into beneficial compounds like short chain fatty acids. A lack of MACs is being looked at as a contributor to inflammation and inflammatory disease (Tan et al., 2014).

moves forward with peristaltic waves that allow food to advance properly from the moment we swallow to the moment we have a bowel movement, except in the cecum. There, the backward waves of peristalsis promote storage and allow bacteria to do what it is supposed to do. Successful FMT occurs when stools are placed directly in the cecum.

Overall, it's estimated that approximately one hundred trillion microscopic organisms inhabit the adult colon and make up the intestinal biome. It is here that bacteria produce enzymes that ferment food into short-chain fatty acids where virus and fungi interfere with pathogens and synthesize vitamins B and K. This is where sh!t happens. It is also where an imbalance of gut flora has been correlated with a host of inflammatory and autoimmune conditions. Diets low in **MACs** (roughage) may increase microbiota that use this mucus barrier as a nutrition source, causing inflammation and leading to leaky gut syndrome (undigested particles leak into the blood stream). Diets low in fiber are also more likely to allow pathogenic bacteria access to our bloodstream.

The cecum's flora also includes low populations of potentially pathogenic micro-organisms such as *Clostridium difficile* or *C. diff.*, which can flourish after antibiotic treatment. *C. diff* is the most common hospital infection in the developed world, causing mild to severe cases of diarrheal illness to life-threatening colitis and toxic megacolon (abnormal dilation of the colon).

Within a month of diagnosis, one out of eleven people over age sixty-five will die of a health-care-associated *C. diff* infection. The infectious rate of *C. diff* has been increasing over the last decade. *C. diff* infection (CDI) costs range from approximately $8,900 to $30,000 for each hospitalized patient—an expense shared by hospitals, third-party payers, and society as a whole, if people are absent from work. Despite increased awareness of the danger of CDI, there is still no consensus on treatment regimens.

Lawsuits have even claimed that hospitals failed to follow safety procedures to prevent *C. diff* and were therefore negligent. However, hospital
sanitation may have nothing to do with outbreaks of *C. diff*.

The solution to the worsening burden of CDI may exist in the intestinal microbiome. There is substantial evidence that fecal microbiota
transplantation (FMT) (the implantation of either a patient's own stool,
known as **autologous transplant**, or healthy donor stool, known as
heterologous transplant) into a patient with a gut microbial imbalance
caused by CDI is a better alternative than traditional antibiotic therapy.
Fecal transplants for recurring *C. diff* have become an accepted life-sav-
ing alternative since 2013 with a 92 percent success rate. The FDA
chose enforcement discretion to "allow" the procedure without formally
approving or disapproving them.

Other common diseases of the large intestine include cancer, polyps
(extra tissue that can become cancerous), ulcerative colitis (ulcers of the
colon and rectum), diverticulitis (inflammation or infection of pouches
in the colon), irritable bowel syndrome (IBS a.k.a. a spastic colon—a
condition causing cramps, bloating, diarrhea or constipation, or both),
and inflammatory bowel disease that includes two chronic inflammatory
conditions: ulcerative colitis (UC) and Crohn's disease (CD). All of these
will be discussed in later chapters.

Excluding skin cancers, **colorectal cancer** is the third most common
cancer in both men and women in the United States, killing over 260,000
lives annually (only lung and bronchial cancer kill more). This is a good
reason for **annual high-sensitivity fecal occult blood tests** (FOBT) and
a colonoscopy if you have blood in your stool, rectal bleeding, or are
more than forty-five years old. Another reason is that this might be your
only opportunity to mail poop to someone without being arrested.

Both polyps and colorectal cancers can bleed, and FOBT checks for
blood in feces (stool) that cannot be seen visually.

RECTUM

After your colon reabsorbs water and electrolytes, the remaining waste is feces or stool, which is stored in the latter part of the large intestine. This part of the large intestine is known as the sigmoid colon, which derives its name from the Greek letter "S" or sigma and attaches to the rectum.

The rectum is a part of the lower gastrointestinal tract about eight inches in length and two and a half inches in diameter at its widest point. The rectum connects to the anus.

Once dried fecal matter or stool (sh!t) accumulates in the sigmoid colon and rectum, if you are lucky, it will eventually cause pressure and you will have the urge to defecate. If you rarely have this inclination, I recommend referring to the chapter in this book about constipation.

An increasingly common problem in the rectum is **proctitis**, a condition in which the lining of the inner rectum becomes inflamed. Proctitis can cause painful straining to defecate, bleeding, or the passage of mucus, and can be a result of Crohn's disease or ulcerative colitis. It can also result from sexually transmitted microbiota like *Neisseria gonorrhoeae* (**gonorrhea**), *Treponema pallidum* (**syphilis**) or the *Herpes simplex* virus (HSV) from anal intercourse.

Proctitis may rarely be caused by *Salmonella*, or by *Clostridium difficile* after antibiotic therapy. It can also be a side effect of radiation treatment.

ANUS

The anus starts at the bottom of the rectum and is where the gastrointestinal tract ends and exits the body. Circular muscles called the external sphincter form the wall of the anus and hold it closed. Glands release fluid to keep it moist.

Hemorrhoids are the most common pain-in-the-ass problems (after spouses). These are swollen veins that may be internal or external. They may result from a number of causes. Pregnancy and straining during

THE SITZ BATH

Start with a clean bathtub or purchase one of the small plastic sitz bath containers made to fit your toilet. Fill with three to four inches of warm water. Some of the small plastic sitz bathtubs come with a bag and a tube for a continuous supply of warm water. Ask your doctor if they recommend adding baking soda or salt. Sit for ten to twenty minutes and then pat dry with a clean towel. This can be done several times a day. Keep your tub clean and rinse well to remove any cleaning chemical residue.

bowel movements are two of the most common. Smaller ones may heal without treatment. Common at-home treatments include: sitz baths (after every bowel movement), small ice packs, witch hazel wipes, hemorrhoid creams containing a local anesthetic, and sitting on a softer surface. Long-term solutions include the increase of fiber, exercise, and water consumption. There are also in-office procedures like rubber band ligation for larger chronic hemorrhoids.

Anal fissures, tears in the lining of the anus, can also cause pain with bowel movements. They are common in infants but can affect people of any age and are often caused by constipation or because of inflammatory bowel disease (IBS). Most anal fissures also get better with simple treatments like increased fiber intake or sitz baths.

A rare condition in the anus parking lot is anal cancer. Infection with **human papillomavirus** (HPV) via anal sex increases the risk. Anal sex also increases the risk of getting anal herpes (HSV-1 and HSC-2). Sufferers usually have painful sores around the anus that come and go.

CONCLUSION

The average transit time through the colon is about forty hours; however, there are significant differences between men and women: thirty-three hours for men compared to forty-seven hours for women (we aren't slow, we're thorough). The whole trip, from chewing to pooing, can take from twenty-four to seventy-two hours.

How often should we poop? Again, there is no such thing as a perfect pooper. Some people poop three times a day and some poop three times a week. If you have pain and bloating combined with small dark stools, you might be constipated, a problem we address in an upcoming chapter.

If your food lingers longer in your stomach, or breakdown is not occurring, food becomes stale. It can begin to decompose and release gas. Think of the whole digestive tract from the stomach to the rectum as a water hose. If at any point in the system something goes wrong, like an opening is not closing or a blockage occurs, the whole system is disrupted. Blockage at any level can alter the normal process and create pressure, gas, distention, and abdominal pain. Good reasons to keep reading.

CHAPTER 4

GAS PRICES

"Let them fart fire and brimstone. I will not have a single case of scurvy on
my hands, the sea-surgeon's shame, while there is cabbage to be culled."
—**Patrick O'Brian's** ***Desolation Island***

The average person passes gas about fourteen times a day whether or
not someone pulls their finger. Intestinal gas is composed mainly of
the odorless gases: hydrogen, nitrogen, and carbon dioxide. Hydrogen sulfide, another component in flatulence, causes it to smell like rotten eggs, but its gaseous cousin, dimethyl sulfide, will impart a sweeter finish resembling a nice port wine. However, about one-third of people have intestinal gas that contains **methane**.

FART LIGHTING—REAL OR URBAN LEGEND?

While not medically sanctioned, according to Thought Co., fart components can ignite. To some extent, you can tell what's in a fart by the flame's color. Orange flames indicate hydrogen while blue indicates methane. (The author does not recommend experimenting with this.)

Methane is mostly produced by the gut bacteria *Methanobrevibacter smithii,* which has been linked to slower small intestinal transit and increased calorie absorption. Because of this, some studies indicate that methane and obesity may be related (Basseri, et al., 2012).

If you have methane in your stool, it will probably float in water. This is not a good experiment for your kid's school science fair, so parents— keep it to yourself.

Researchers (Manichanh et al., 2014) who measure flatulence (via gas collection balloon catheters) have found that people who complain about gas symptoms do fart more often, but no more total volume than their healthy non-complaining counterparts. Thus, advancing the conclusions that:

1. Researchers lead interesting lives
2. People who are willing to volunteer as research subjects are true heroes.

The Manichanh research team also found marked evidence of microbial dysbiosis in the group who complained about flatulence. Although the microbiota of the healthy group and the complaining group were similar in main bacterial families, there were notable differences between the groups in the smaller bacterial families. In conclusion they noted, "Patients complaining of flatulence have a poor tolerance of intestinal gas, which is associated with the microbial ecosystem."

But gas is not always a sign of poor digestive health or microbial imbalance. It is simply an inconvenience, especially if you're stuck in an elevator. The best digestive advice I can give most people (even those in the elevator) is keep it movin' with fiber and exercise. It's the slower gut that usually has bacterial overgrowth. If you suspect that you have abnormal gassiness, you should see a doctor. No one wants to live with a human whoopee cushion.

Sometimes gassiness can come on quickly. People who are **lactose intolerant** may become gassy about thirty minutes after consuming milk products. However, a good rule of thumb is that it takes six to eight hours for a particular food to produce gas, but certain combinations may speed up or slow down the process. For anyone who cracked up over the flatulence scene in *Blazing Saddles*—it was probably beans from the previous meal that made it a musical.

Gassy foods are always a popular topic with GI doctors. We all have our list of foods that make it challenging to be around us, but the fact is that everyone processes food differently. What is gigantically gassy for some, may do nothing to others. It's individual genetics along with our biomes and hormones that make our farts special.

BEANS

Legumes are probably the most notorious gas producers. However, the little toots are protein and nutrient dense and a good source of fiber!

Now that I've used the f-word, I'll just say it: adults need twenty-five to thirty-eight grams of fiber every day (See p. 54 for more fiber info). Navy beans have ten grams of fiber per half-cup cooked serving—eat up. Pinto beans and black beans are both rich in carbs, protein, and fiber while being low in fat. You get satiety (that full feeling), fiber, and flatulence all in one food.

One reason that beans produce gas is that they contain raffinose and oligosaccharides which are gas-producing sugars found in many vegetables. The best way to decrease their gas production is to let the dried beans soak in cold water for eight hours, pour off the water, and cook in fresh water.

CHICKPEAS A.K.A. GARBANZO BEANS

Hummus is a popular Mediterranean food but extremely gassy because of its main ingredient: the chickpea. Like beans, chickpeas have similar problems when it comes to being digested in the stomach, even though their health benefits are great. If you still want to enjoy chickpeas and their health benefits, you should soak them in water for ten to fifteen hours before cooking.

When boiling the chickpeas, it's a good idea to scrape off the layer of foam that appears at the top of the pot. You might toss a bay leaf into the pot if your stomach is more sensitive. Many people claim that bay leaves aid them in digestion. And while hummus is popular at group events, consider forgoing it at Superbowl parties since you might not get out before the flatulence sets in.

ARTICHOKES

This meaty thistle is a good source of dietary fiber, folate, and vitamins C and K. Packed with antioxidants, artichokes are ranked number seven on the USDA's top twenty antioxidant-rich foods list. Have you ever eaten the steamed artichoke at The Cheesecake Factory?

One can probably get away with eating a single artichoke, but after the second one you'll most likely feel extremely gassy. Why? Because artichokes contain a significant amount of fructans, an indigestible fiber. If you love artichokes but want to play it safe, the canned variety don't seem to be as gassy because of the liquid and preservatives they sit in for months at a time. More artichoke info later in the Money in the Bank chapter.

BEER

Beer is one of the oldest drinks in history. Chemical tests of ancient pottery jars reveal that beer was produced as far back as about seven thousand years ago. There is even a receipt for beer on stone dating back to 2050 BC from the Sumerian city of Umma in ancient Iraq. Go to Wikipedia, "History of Beer" for photo.

Beer drinkers may experience flatulence and bloating for more than one reason. Beer is carbonated, which means those bubbles may accumulate in your gut. According to the American College of Gastroenterology, "Moderate Alcohol Consumption is Associated with Small Intestinal Bacterial Overgrowth." When the charts of 198 patients who underwent lactulose hydrogen breath testing (LHBT) to determine the presence of small intestinal bacterial overgrowth (SIBO) researchers found that alcohol consumption was significantly associated with the presence of SIBO. One of the hallmark symptoms of SIBO is excess gas.

CORN

Corn may be a vegetable whose only purpose is to make oil. The best thing I can say to a bite of corn is, "See ya later." Because if you eat a corn kernel, chances are you will soon find that same unchanged kernel in your poop. It has a low nutritional content, serves no benefits in digestion, and has been over-genetically modified. As a society, we have been conditioned to eat popcorn at the movies, corn on the cob at dinner, or corn casseroles on Thanksgiving. Some people think that corn is a nutritional vegetable that nourishes their bodies. The unfortunate reality is that corn has few absorbable vitamins or minerals. Even if corn doesn't make you gassy, the wear and tear on your digestive process isn't worth the trouble.

SALADS

All green vegetables in general can cause gas, especially when eaten raw. The raw movement has been in full swing since the 1970s, but for people with digestive challenges, eating raw contributes to bloating, indigestion, constipation or loose stools, weight gain, malnutrition, food allergies, and a lowered immune system. Digesting raw foods requires more energy and causes more wear and tear on the GI tract. Many of us just can't digest some of the fiber in raw vegetables.

Eating raw can also feed the bacteria in your gut and more bacteria means more gas. Unless you are a rabbit, try cutting back on salads and see if your digestion improves.

NUTS

Because of the high fat and fiber content in nuts, it takes a while for them to be properly digested. As they spend a lot of time working through the digestive system, the risk for gas and bloating is significant.

For a long time, it's been said that nuts should

> **Diverticulosis** occurs when small, bulging pouches (diverticula) form in the digestive tract. When these pouches become inflamed or infected, the condition is called diverticulitis. Nuts and seeds are known to irritate diverticula in some people.

be avoided by people with diverticulosis or pockets in the colon. Recent studies show that nuts protect against heart disease, but like any food you put into your body, you should look at your risk vs. benefit ratio. For example, if you're a patient with diverticular disease who's unlikely to develop heart disease—but far more likely to perforate your colon by eating nuts—the choice is simple. If your colon is intact and free of these pockets, but your heart attack risk is more substantial due to high occurrences in family history or high cholesterol, then eat nuts.

DAIRY

Dairy foods become a problem if you're lactose intolerant. Lactose is the natural sugar that's found in milk. It's also found in most common milk products, such as cheese, ice cream, and many processed foods. Some people—particularly those of Native American, African, or Asian descent—have low levels of the lactase enzyme needed to digest lactose.

> ## SYMPTOMS OF LACTOSE INTOLERANCE:
> - Abdominal bloating, pain, or cramps
> - Borborygmi (rumbling or gurgling from the stomach)
> - Diarrhea
> - Flatulence
> - Nausea and/or Vomiting

Other people can eat cheese, but not sour cream. The hydrogen breath test (HBT) after consumption of lactose is currently considered the best way to diagnose lactose intolerance due to its sensitivity, its simplicity, its low cost, and non-invasiveness.

Most people who are lactose intolerant can eat small amounts of dairy in order to get their daily requirements of calcium. Some can tolerate cheese while others can eat yogurt.

Some dairy, like yogurt, is marketed as healthy. However, flavored yogurts with added sugars can be high in carbs that feed bad bacteria and cause gas and bloating in people who are not usually lactose intolerant.

The research team of Fassio, Facioni, and Guagnini (2018) concluded that lactose intolerant people *should* avoid foods containing lactose. However, the main therapeutic intervention for lactose-intolerant people is the administration of lactase as a food supplement. In addition to lactase, specific strains of probiotics that express β-galactosidase activity will also improve tolerance.

TOMATOES, EGGPLANTS, AND BELL PEPPERS

Plants in the nightshade family such as tomatoes, eggplant, potatoes, and bell peppers are generally thought to be an important part of a healthy diet, but one key ingredient in all of these foods has the potential to cause serious gut issues. Naturally occurring **glycoalkaloids** (a bitter compound that can cause burning when eaten) found in all nightshades can cause nightshade intolerance. Glycoalkaloids have been shown to lead to intestinal inflammation and the condition known as "leaky gut" in mice. In the case of the bell pepper, the smooth skin needs bile from the gall bladder in order to be digested. Because of this method of digestion, more gas is produced.

BREADS AND PASTAS

Gluten is a protein found in a number of grains such as wheat and barley. The last two decades have shown that an increase in gluten intolerance leads to celiac sprue, also known as celiac disease (page 102). Celiac sprue is defined as a disease involving damage to the villi of the small intestine. Over time, repeated exposure to gluten destroy villi. For some, avoiding gluten can be the difference between life and death. But other studies (Catassi, et al., 2016; Volta, Caio, Tovoli, & De Giorgio, 2013; Sapone et al., 2012) have found that gluten can trigger stomach pain, bloating, and fatigue

SOME SYMPTOMS OF NIGHTSHADE INTOLERANCE:

- Acid reflux
- Arthritis
- Breathing difficulties
- Diarrhea
- Heartburn
- Irritable bowels
- Itching
- Joint pain
- Leaky gut
- Mouth swelling (rare)
- Swelling in the joints

Villi in the small intestine are small finger-like projections of tissue that increase the surface area of the intestine and contain specialized cells that transport substances into the bloodstream and help with nutrient absorption.

even in those without the disease. This has become known as **non-celiac gluten sensitivity** (**NCGS**). If you think breads and pastas may be causing your stomach problems, try going gluten-free. Some notice improvement in weeks, but for the especially gluten sensitive it may take six months for the intestines to normalize.

OATMEAL

I always find it interesting when previously asymptomatic patients come in with symptoms of excessive gas. Usually, within the first minute or two, they tell me they've decided to change their diets to what advertisers call, "Slim up for summer!" Inevitably, this gas victim is on a new diet that's high in oatmeal. In fact, 20 percent of people who had never eaten oats find that they are actually allergic to them. I can't count how many times I've heard, "But doctor, I read that oatmeal is good for you." My answer is always: "Yes, oats can be good for some people, but not you." It is oatmeal's high amount of soluble fiber that causes the gassiness in some people.

BROCCOLI, CAULIFLOWER, AND BRUSSEL SPROUTS

All cruciferous vegetables can cause gas. Cauliflower, cabbage, garden cress, bok choy, broccoli, Brussels sprouts, and kale, while nutrient-rich, are notorious gas producers due to their fiber and raffinose—a sugar that

---

SYMPTOMS OF NCGS THAT USUALLY CLOSELY FOLLOW EATING GLUTEN AND DISAPPEAR AFTER GLUTEN WITHDRAWAL:

- Abdominal pain
- Altered bowel habits
- Bloating
- Bone or joint pain
- Fatigue
- Hair loss
- Headache
- Mood disorders
- Rashes or eczema

remains undigested until microbes in your gut ferment it, which produces gas. But cooking tends to reduce their flatulent potential. Roast, steam, grill, do what you will!

SORBITOL

Yep, the sweet in Sweet-N-Low may make for not-so-sweet flatulence. Just like fructose, sorbitol can cause an increase in gas if ingested excessively. Sorbitol is a sugar alcohol that can have a laxative effect by drawing water into the bowels. Though it occurs naturally in some fruits—like apples, peaches, and prunes—it's found mainly as an artificial sweetener in candies and gum.

WHIP IT

The swallowing of air or **aerophagia** is common among bottle-fed infants and adolescent boys learning to burp on command, but it can lead to gas. Beware of whipped foods like malts and shakes. All that air has to go somewhere. The carbonation and sugars in fizzy beverages like sodas can also cause gas as can carbonated water. Even healthy, blended smoothies cause problems for some. Smokers and some gum chewers are more likely to suffer from aerophagia resulting in bloating, belching, and flatulence.

THE SOLUTIONS

Most flatulence can be lessened by avoiding the foods that trigger it. Cooking, especially steaming, can reduce many foods' flatulent potential. Drinking liquids thirty minutes before a meal instead of while you are eating also helps some. Chewing well and eating slower may reduce swallowed air and improve digestion.

The **parasympathetic** nervous system is the part of the autonomic (involuntary) nervous system that controls functions of the body at rest. The parasympathetic system slows heart rate, increases intestinal and gland activity, and relaxes muscles in the gastrointestinal tract. The **sympathetic** nervous system is the part of the autonomic nervous system that prepares the body to react to stresses like threats or injuries.

As a general rule, the best digestive advice I can offer is to sit, chew your food, and focus on eating. Do not get up from a meal and go running. Exercise creates discord between your sympathetic and parasympathetic nervous system, causing chaos in your gut.

Parsley is an herb also known to reduce gas and bloating. The ancient Egyptians referred to it as "mountain celery" and used it to combat stomach pains. It is also a diuretic and helps to remove water and salt from the body. It can be added to steeping tea or chewed raw. I have also known patients who've had success with **chamomile, peppermint,** and **cinnamon** teas for gas. However, everyone is different and occasionally these teas can even cause stomach distress.

My favorite go-to for reducing gas is **fennel**. My own experience has found this aromatic, licorice-like herb to be quite versatile. The entire plant is edible. The stalks can be added to fish and vegetable stock. The top part or fronds can be a garnish, added to salads, or made into pesto or even fennel butter.

It lowers gas production and can be consumed in food or made into a tea. Because it does not have any laxative effects, it can be eaten at any time. The Bulgarian researchers (Chakŭrski, Matev, Koĭchev, &

Angelova, 1981) successfully used fennel in combination with dandelion and St. John's wort to treat patients with chronic non-specific colitis.

FENNEL SALAD REMEDY

- Lemon juice
- Fresh fennel bulbs (remove tough outer layers and shave or cut into thin slices.
- Fennel fronds
- Preserved lemons
- Olive oil

CHAPTER 5

NO SH!T

"I wish that being famous helped me from being constipated."
—**Marvin Gaye**

While keeping some things to yourself is a good idea, clogged plumbing—whether it's in your house or in your abdomen—is bad. How do you know if you are constipated? Once again, everyone is different.

Do you have a full feeling that does not go away several hours after eating? Is pooping painful for you? Do you push and strain? Do you have pencil-like poop? Or perhaps you poop small, hard, round pebbles. If you answered yes to any of the above questions, it probably means:

1. You spend too much time analyzing poop.
2. You are constipated. But keep in mind, some of us are daily poopers, and some of us feel lucky to poop twice a week. Everyone is different. Even those who poop several times a day are rarely unhealthy.

Because constipation is such a common problem, affecting as much as 80 percent of the population at one time or another, doctors developed the

Meyers Scale (a.k.a. Bristol Scale) to help patients describe their poop without bringing in colored photos. If your poop is a three or four on the scale, the poop fairy has blessed you. If it is a one or two, you may be constipated and the wicked stitch witch has sent in the flying monkeys—prepare for cramps.

MEYERS STOOL SCALE

1. Pebble-like, small, round, hard to pass
2. Sausage-shaped, lumpy
3. Sausage-shaped with surface cracks
4. Sausage or snake-like but smooth and soft
5. Soft separate blobs, easy to pass
6. Fluffy, mushy
7. Watery

Numbers five, six, or seven usually indicate the diarrhea devil. I know what you are thinking: there should be a lot more categories! What about those hard-to-pass blobs that look like Silly-Putty? And those mucous covered popcorn-like poops?

But what is normal for you? If your poop has looked like silly putty your whole life and you don't experience any pain, this could be your normal. All I'm saying is that *normal* is a relative term. After all, wombats have cube-shaped feces. But if pooping is often painful, you may have chronic constipation.

Women, because of the extra internal organs like ovaries and uterus, have slightly longer, more winding colons (**tortuous colons**) and are more prone to constipation than men who have more muscle strength to push food

News you can use: A **tortuous colon** has an excessive number of sharp bends. A **redundant colon** has an excessive number of loops. Neither one is unhealthy, but can make a colonoscopy more challenging.

> **Endometriosis** is the growth of endometrial tissue outside of the uterus. **Endometrial** tissue consists of glands, blood cells, and connective tissue that normally grows in the uterus, to prepare the lining of the womb for ovulation. They can develop anywhere in the body but usually occur in the pelvis.

through. Women, for the most part, have tortuous colons from pregnancy. The effect of a uterus squeezing the bowels for nine months and then pushing a baby out creates a roller coaster in the bowels that is sometimes resistant to correction. In fact, after two or three pregnancies, most women will have bowel problems.

Bowel tortuosity can also be the result of scar tissue forming after abdominal or pelvic surgery, or even a condition called **endometriosis**. Endometriosis can cause abnormal tissue to deposit around the bowels causing a phenomenon of pseudo-obstruction which would present as constipation.

Endometriosis and scar tissue of the bowels are not easy to diagnose and are a diagnosis of exclusion. They can be quite debilitating and may cause obstructions or pseudo-obstructions in the future. Obstructions of the bowels can eventually require surgery. Pseudo-obstruction rarely requires a surgical solution.

> **Intestinal pseudo-obstruction** is a result of nerve or muscle problems that prevent the intestines from contracting normally to move food, fluid, and air through the intestines. Symptoms may include cramps, abdominal pain, nausea, vomiting, bloating, constipation, and occasionally diarrhea.

The older we get the more likely we are to suffer from constipation. Acute constipation can block the intestine, which may even require surgery. But you can take a deep, statistical breath because research has found no link between constipation and colorectal cancers.

> ## SIGNS YOU MIGHT NEED A COLONOSCOPY:
> - Abnormal weight loss
> - Anemia
> - Change/pain in bowel habits from normal
> - Rectal bleeding

Research has shown that anyone with a change in bowel movements needs to see a doctor. If you go from normal to constipated, you should definitely consult a gastroenterologist.

The contributing factors for constipation are about as long as the small intestine itself.

Constipation is more common among the poor, the depressed, the sedentary, the dense urban dwellers, and the physically and/or sexually abused. About 25 percent of those chronically constipated have biological relatives who also report chronic constipation (Forootan, Bagheri, & Darvishi, 2018).

Other factors include: low-fiber diets, low fluid intake, hormone imbalances (including thyroid, progesterone, and estrogen), medications, failing to respond to the urge to defecate, irritable bowel syndrome, abnormalities of the anatomy, reduced motility of the large intestine (slow transit constipation or **STC** caused by abnormalities of the enteric nerves), and my favorite: **idiopathic constipation**—no known cause. Although I feel "no known cause" is usually lack of detective work from a healthcare system that supports insurance companies more than patients or doctors.

One common denominator that I warn people about is chocolate. One little bite of chocolate is like swallowing mortar for some and can mean a week without poop.

MEDICATIONS THAT CAN CAUSE CONSTIPATION:

- Antacids, especially those with calcium and aluminum
- Anti-cholinergic agents like atropine, trihexyphenidyl
- Anticonvulsants like phenytoin, clonazepam
- Antidiarrheal agents like loperamide and attapulgite
- Antihistamines like diphenhydramine
- Anti-Parkinson's drugs like Levodopa
- Antipsychotics like clozapine, thioridazine, Achlorpromazine
- Antispasmodics like dicyclomine
- Calcium supplements
- Calcium channel blockers such as verapamil
- Diuretics for heart failure like furosemide
- High blood pressure drugs like methyldopa, clonidine, apropranolol, etc.
- Iron supplements
- Opioid pain relievers like morphine, codeine etc.
- Oral contraceptives
- Pain relievers or NSAIDs like ibuprofen and aspirin
- Terbutaline used for bronchial asthma
- Tricyclic antidepressants like amitriptyline
- Sympathomimetics like ephedrine and terbutaline
- Miscellaneous compounds including Octreotide used in medical imaging; polystyrene resins used to remove ions such as potassium, calcium, and sodium from solutions in technical or medical applications; and cholestyramine for lowering cholesterol

WHAT ARE FECES?

Feces are what is left after the nutrients have been absorbed from food. Feces are about 75 percent water, bacteria (living and dead), and undigested fiber and protein. You can see why not enough liquid or fiber might slow down the whole procession.

Feces also contains small amounts of cells, mucus, salt, and fat. Feces are usually brown because of bile and the breakdown of red blood cells during the digestive process. Humans excrete about twenty-five thousand pounds of poop in an average lifetime or about three hundred pounds a year and have several pounds of feces in their digestive tract at any given time. So, when someone says, "You're full of it!" they are correct.

COLONIC INERTIA A.K.A. SLOW TRANSIT CONSTIPATION

You don't see the corn you ate on Monday until the following weekend. And when your first-degree biological relatives get together, they all agree: "Constipation is the family curse." While *corn tracers* are a common-sense approach, there is a diagnostic procedure that uses either a wireless motility capsule (**WMC**) or a radiopaque capsule (marker) instead of corn.

The radiopaque marker is most commonly used. The marker's progress is followed through the digestive tract using X-rays.

The WMC uses radionuclide scintigraphy, not to be confused with cinematography (no one gets an Oscar).

The WMC can relay much more information than the radiopaque marker. It tracks your temperature and pH throughout your whole digestive process and downloads it to a data receiver that you wear. It can diagnose gastroparesis (slow-emptying stomach) as well as track small and large intestine transit time.

You return the radio receiver (not the capsule) to the gastroenterologist who downloads the information and analyzes it.

Colonic inertia is a severe, unrelenting constipation with abdominal distention and pain. Individuals with colonic inertia often do not pass a stool for seven to ten days at a time and sometimes longer. Sometimes colonic inertia is accompanied by motility problems of the upper intestine including delayed emptying of the stomach (gastroparesis) and small intestinal pseudo-obstruction (symptoms of blockage, but no actual blockage).

There is a less expensive test that I call "the ring study." Not to be confused with jewelry shopping—a radiologist will have you swallow a radiopaque (shows on X-rays) plastic ring then take X-ray images on day four, day seven, and day ten after swallowing to chart its movement.

CURES?

Laxatives are okay for the occasional bout of constipation but as a daily or even weekly remedy, they are stressing your digestive tract and the trillions of microbes that live there. Fasting and starving is associated with increased *Akkermansia muciniphila* bacterium (Sonoyama, et al., 2009; Remely, et al., 2015). *A. muciniphila* in increased numbers has also been linked to certain types of colon cancer (Zackular et al., 2013). However, others disagree about the role of *Akkermansia muciniphila* in the colon. (More research is needed to define the role of bacteria in disease.)

Laxatives are never a good idea for the long term or for weight loss. Most calories are absorbed by the small intestine, and laxatives act on the large intestine and do not aid in weight loss, only waste loss. Laxatives can also cause electrolyte and mineral (zinc, potassium, sodium, and chloride) imbalances, dehydration, chronic constipation that can lead to laxative dependence, and even kidney failure.

Laxatives like senna will stimulate bowel evacuation that otherwise would not occur for days. Then your colon muscles will stop moving because they have nothing to do. Like any muscle that is not in use, colon muscles atrophy (weaken), which slows digestion, making you want to take another laxative and the whole cycle begins again.

I have seen several colons that have lost elasticity due to laxatives. They behave like a rough piece of leather. This can lead to a complete colon resection where the damaged portion of the colon has to be removed.

Sometimes, the two ends of the colon or rectum cannot be reattached. Then a procedure known as a colostomy has to be performed where an opening is made on the outside of

NOT ALL LAXATIVES ARE CREATED EQUAL:

- Stimulant laxatives like **Senokot** and **Ex-Lax** are brand names of senna, a natural vegetable laxative that causes the intestines to contract and push stool out.
- Bulk-forming laxatives create softer, easy-to-pass stools. They include **Metamucil** (psyllium), **Fibercon** (polycarbophil), and **Citrucel** (methylcellulose).
- Osmotic laxatives like **MiraLAX** and **Milk of Magnesia** increase water in the stool, making it softer and easier to pass.
- Stool softeners like **Colace** (docusate sodium and docusate calcium) decrease the surface tension of stools so that they absorb more water, making them softer.
- Special use laxatives include lubricant laxatives (decrease water in the intestine), saline laxatives (pre-op), and prokinetic laxatives (IBS).

the body so that one end of the bowel can excrete feces into an attached colostomy bag. An early diagnosis for the cause of constipation can save some patients from this life-changing procedure.

EAT MORE FIBER?

If you suffer from slow transit constipation, there's a chance that no amount of fiber betting will produce a jackpot. It could even cause the constipation to worsen.

Research (Ho, Tan, Daud, & Seow-Choen, 2018) found that patients with idiopathic constipa-

> **FOODS I RECOMMEND AVOIDING IF YOU SUFFER FROM CONSTIPATION:**
> - Apples
> - Bananas
> - Chocolate
> - Rice
> - White bread

tion improved after reducing or eliminating all types of fiber from their diet. Other research has found varying outcomes, depending on what type of fiber was introduced.

TYPES OF FIBER

There are two types of fiber: **soluble** and **insoluble**. Both fibers are plant-based carbohydrates. Soluble or digestible fiber attracts water and turns to mush (chyme) during digestion. Many foods contain both types of fiber. Soluble fiber is found in apricots, avocados, beans (black, navy, and kidney), barley, broccoli, Brussels sprouts, figs, lentils, peas, pears, nectarines, nuts, oat bran/oatmeal, seeds, soybeans, sweet potatoes, and turnips. It's also found in psyllium, a common fiber supplement like Metamucil. Soluble fiber slows digestion and allows more nutrient absorption. Some types of soluble fiber may help lower the risk of heart disease.

Insoluble or indigestible fiber does not dissolve. It remains more or less unchanged as it moves through the digestive tract. There is evidence that indicates dietary fibers modulate intestinal microbiota by stimulating beneficial bacteria and suppressing pathogenic (bad) bacteria (Chen et al., 2013).

Because it is not digested at all, insoluble fiber is not a source of calories but fills up space in the stomach and intestines, giving us the sensation of fullness. It adds bulk to the stool and appears to help food pass through our digestive tract more quickly. Insoluble fiber is found in wheat bran, whole-wheat bread, brown rice, the skins of fruit, coconut, flax seeds, lentils, nuts, okra, turnips, green beans, potato skins, cauliflower, and corn.

You may need to experiment with different types of fiber-rich foods to figure out if your constipation is from a lack of fiber. We are all different. What is perfume for one person may be poison to another.

I always recommend people start by eating sweet potatoes. Baked or mashed, sweet potatoes are rich in fiber and easy to prepare.

Consider eating prunes. Dried plums (prunes) have both kinds of fiber plus they contain sorbitol, which has a natural, laxative effect. In a 2011 study by Attaluri, Donahoe, Valestin, Brown, and Rao, forty constipated subjects found that fifty grams of prunes twice daily with meals were as effective as psyllium in relieving constipation. This comes to a total of about ten to twelve prunes per day. My advice is to start with fewer prunes and increase slowly until you get the desired results. A word of caution: never begin your prune journey less than twenty-four hours before a trans-Atlantic plane ride or a long hike.

FYI, dark chocolate trumps prunes. If you eat dark chocolate with prunes . . . chocolate will win. Prepare for constipation.

FATS

In 2010, an article in *the European Journal of Clinical Nutrition* cited research by Clegg et al. (2011) who found an increase in gastric emptying when subjects consumed a high-fat diet. Fats! Say it ain't so. You've done so well on that low-fat diet. What you have to remember is that some fats are healthier than others.

Monounsaturated fats and **polyunsaturated fats** (omega-3 and omega-6) are known as good fats. Avocadoes, nuts, fish, sunflower seeds, plant-based oils like canola oil, olive oil, safflower oil, sunflower oil, sesame oil, peanut oil, and peanut butter are all considered good fat foods. Yes, you may use the words "good" and "fat" in the same sentence.

Another form of good fat is **medium-chain triglycerides** or MCTs. Research has shown that MCTs play a role in lowering weight, decreasing metabolic syndrome, abdominal obesity, and inflammation. MCTs are abundant in most forms of coconut (except coconut water) and palm kernel oil, according to the US Department of Agriculture National Nutrient Database. Palm kernel oil is recently undergoing scrutiny for its high saturated fats and may not be a good choice for those with heart disease.

HERBS

There are certain herbs that have been used through the ages for constipation. Yellow dock (*Rumex crispus*) has been known to relieve constipation. Both the leaves and root may have a mild laxative effect. Use the leaves from a young plant and boil in several changes of water before consuming.

RECTAL SENSORIMOTOR DYSFUNCTION

There are some constipation issues that are related more to mechanical and anatomical problems than to diet, hormones, or lifestyle. Rectal examinations are usually conducted before more extensive testing if these types of problems are suspected. Using a gloved finger, doctors perform an intrarectal examination and can evaluate the muscle tone of the rectum and feel any weakening between the rectum and the pelvic floor. While this may be one of the least favorite of all medical tests, in the end, it's necessary.

Using a flexible scope via a sigmoidoscopy or colonoscopy, doctors can look for possible causes of unexplained symptoms. An **anorectal manometry** (ARM—it's not what you think) examination might also be useful. This procedure uses a pressure sensitive balloon-tipped catheter to measure the nerve and muscle capacity of the anus and rectum. An ARM is used to diagnose problematic desire-to-defecate thresholds, which are usually a failure of nerve and muscle coordination.

Another test, the **balloon expulsion test** (BET), measures the amount of time needed to expel an air- or water-filled rectal balloon. Patients who can then twist the balloon into the shape of a Dachshund get a discount in my office.

A long-standing diagnostic procedure is the lower gastrointestinal series or **barium enema**. Barium is a metallic substance that is radiopaque (appears solid on an X-ray). These X-rays can reveal details surrounding many physical abnormalities. Afterward, you may need a laxative or enema, and then prepare to poop white bricks.

Barium is also used in defecography and magnetic resonance defecography (MRD), which create an image of the rectum and pelvic floor. The barium is imaged as it leaves the rectum tracking any abnormal functioning.

> The **CT** or **computerized tomography**, also called the CAT scan, is medical imagining that uses computers and rotating X-ray machines to create detailed cross section images of tissue, bone, and blood vessels.

What are **probiotics**?
Microbes assumed to be good for us are grown in a liquid (usually milk) then processed in ways to make them live longer. Research results on the efficacy of probiotic therapy have been inconsistent. However, not all probiotics are created equal. Some of them are no more than snake oil.

Lastly, the CT scan may be necessary to determine if constipation is due to obstructions caused by the pressure of other organs on the colon. I have seen many ovarian tumors present as constipation.

Playing detective with your symptoms may lead to a consultation with a gastroenterologist. Remember, always go to the doctor if your constipation is new or if you have rectal bleeding.

MORE SOLUTIONS

According to the American Gastroenterological Association, 70 percent of all patients with gastrointestinal disorders improve after **biofeedback therapy**. This is done by placing a probe into the anus that monitors the patient tensing their muscles on a computer screen. Biofeedback therapy has been used quite successfully to improve constipation due to rectal dysfunction by coordinating the muscles and nerves involved with defecation. Perhaps patients just claim to get better so they don't have to attend more probing sessions. Either way, someone checks the box.

A review of **probiotics** for the treatment of chronic constipation demonstrated that certain probiotics did cause a significant improvement in the number of stools per week (Dimidi, Christodoulides, Fragkos, Scott, & Whelan, 2014). Several reasons have been proposed to account for this improvement:

1. Probiotics may alter the intestinal microbiota.

2. Probiotic metabolites may act as promotility agents.
3. Probiotics may change the pH of the lining of the intestines and reduce inflammation (Waller et al., 2011).

Occasionally, **surgery** is recommended for chronic constipation, especially for those who have abused laxatives. For many years, colon surgical resections were considered an option. Now, less invasive procedures like **sacral nerve modulation** (SNM) are more likely. SNM is the implantation of a permanent electrical stimulation device that *encourages* the neural pathways involved in defecation and/or bladder function.

A growing body of research suggests that dysbiosis may be the cause of chronic constipation.

PRESCRIPTION OPTIONS FOR CHRONIC CONSTIPATION:

- Lubiprostone is a fatty acid capsule for long-term therapy.
- Linaclotide increases intestinal fluids, helps with pain, bloating, and stool consistency.
- Colchicine is an alkaloid used as a gut anti-inflammatory.
- Alvimopan is used for post-surgical opioid-induced constipation, but can have serious cardiovascular side effects. For short-term use only.
- Vancomycin is an antibiotic used to treat colitis after antibiotic therapy. It only treats bacterial infections in the intestines.

Researchers (Kirgizov, Sukhorukov, Dudarev, & Istomin, 2001 and Gerritsen, Smidt, Rijkers, & de Vos, 2011) found decreases in the bacteria *Lactobacillus*, *Bifidobacterium*, and *Bacteroides spp.* correlated with parallel increases in the potentially pathogenic microorganisms *Pseudomonas aeruginosa* and *Campylobacter jejuni* in constipated subjects.

Khalif, Quigley, Konovitch, and Maximova (2005) also reported decreased levels of *Bifidobacteria* and *Lactobacillus* in adult patients with constipation.

A pediatric study (Zoppi, Cinquetti, Luciano, Benini, Muner, & Minelli, 1998) indicated that *Clostridia* and *Bifidobacteria* were significantly increased in constipated children and the *clostridium* species from constipated children were different from those from healthy controls.

Scientists (Zhu et al., 2014) observed a significant decrease in *Prevotella* and increased representation in several genera of *Firmicutes* in constipated patients compared with controls.

Lactobacillus reuteri has also increased bowel movement frequency in both adult and pediatric patients with constipation (Wu et al., 2013). Additional evidence showed *L. reuteri* could promote both the frequency and velocity of colon neuromuscular activity between meals (Barbara et al., 2005).

In 2018, Japanese researchers Ohara and Suzutani implanted donor microbiota into an eighty-three-year-old male patient who had suffered with chronic constipation for fifty years. Included in the research paper was that he also had symptoms of mild dementia that caused forgetfulness. Was he really constipated or simply forgot the last time he pooped?

The subject was examined for any diseases that might have caused the constipation. None were found. The transplant was infused via colonoscopy into the cecum.

In short, bowel movements were improved and increases in transplanted microbes, particularly *Bifidobacterium* and *Clostridium were seen.*

Published online in *Clinical Case Reports (2018)*, "This beneficial effect of FMT therapy may be applicable for other diseases, such as diabetes mellitus, inflammatory bowel disease, and dementia. We plan to perform a full analysis of the incorporated microbes in a further study."

Ohara and Suzutani's approach for chronic constipation may answer questions like, "Is FMT safe?" and "Will it work?" but we need more. How long will one FMT correct constipation? Will recipients need multiple transplants? Should we be looking for donor feces high in the *Bifidobacterium* and *Clostridium* genera? Or is a richer range of bacteria needed? Do particular species of Bifidobacterium and Clostridium work better than others? Are there long-term effects?

> **FMT** or fecal microbiota transplant is the transfer of feces from a healthy donor into a recipient in order to restore the bacterial balance of the recipient (see p. 125).

Answers to these questions stemming from the exciting research of Dr. Thomas Borody (our content editor) are on the horizon. I consider Dr. Borody the father of modern FMT and a true pioneer who has shone a bright light on the microbiome. Thanks to him we have great expectations for the future.

I have come to think of our microbiome as a garden. And, as every gardener knows, occasionally weeds take over and flowers die. Think of FMT as springtime in the intestine. Time to pull weeds, fertilize, and plant new flowers.

CHAPTER 6

INFURIATING BLOODY DIARRHEA

"I have lived most my life with chronic inflammation
and constant pain with immediate diarrhea."
—Mike McCready, lead guitarist for Pearl Jam

nflammatory bowel disease includes two chronic inflammatory conditions: ulcerative colitis (UC) and Crohn's disease (CD). Much like
cable TV prices, **inflammatory bowel disease** (IBD) is on the rise.
Roughly 1.4 million people in the US and 2.2 million in Europe suffer
from IBD (much lower than the fifty million who pay for cable TV). It is
believed that increased urban living (Soon et al., 2012) may play a role in
the explosion of IBD rates, which doubled in several twentieth-century
decades.

Historically, Asia has had lower IBD rates, but is currently also see-
ing an increase. In Hong Kong the age-adjusted incidence of IBD has
increased from 0.1 per one hundred thousand in 1985 to more than
three per one hundred thousand in 2014. Japan has over two hundred
thousand cases of IBD. Korea, Taiwan, and China have also shown an

increase (Ng, Siew C., 2016). These increases are also believed to be due to an increase in urbanization. Urbanization is associated with a more-westernized diet, antibiotic use, hygiene status, microbial exposures, and pollution.

ULCERATIVE COLITIS

Ulcerative colitis is typically characterized by continuous mucosal inflammation of the rectum and colon causing bloody diarrhea. UC patients usually report pain, urgency, inability to defecate (despite overwhelming urgency), weight loss, and fatigue. Chuck Lorre, the American King of sitcoms, once wrote that having ulcerative colitis made him "appreciative of the life-affirming qualities in a good bowel movement." We can all agree that regularity is appreciated. Yes, even those of us who are not rich and famous have learned this.

CROHN'S DISEASE

Burrill Crohn first described this disease in 1932. CD is spotty inflammation that can be observed in any portion of the GI tract (from mouth to anus). Crohn's also causes diarrhea which can be bloody. Crohn's patients may have fevers, nausea, body aches, weight loss, fatigue, and occasional eye pain. Many patients have symptoms for years before they are diagnosed.

Bowel obstructions due to Crohn's inflammation are common. Tobacco smokers are twice as likely to develop CD as non-smokers, but males and females are affected equally.

Recent next-generation sequencing of intestinal microbes has found that Crohn's is a multifactorial disease.

Some Crohn's sufferers have been found to have excess *Proteus mirabilis*. The Proteus genus is commonly associated with urinary tract infections but has only recently been associated with Crohn's symptoms.

Proteus belong to the *Enterobacteriaceae* family and are common in the gastrointestinal microbiota (Hamilton, Kamm, Ng, & Morrison, 2018).

Another bacterium, *Mycobacterium avium* subspecies *paratuberculosis* (MAP) has also been suspected in Crohn's (Agrawal, G., Borody, T.J.; Chamberlin, W., 2014; Zhou et al., 2016; and Kuenstner, et al., 2017). Many Crohn's disease patients have an immune system that does not allow their macrophages to recognize and control MAP. An increase in *Enterococcus faecalis* bacterium is also associated with Crohn's.

There is more! Patients with Crohn's disease have also been found to have a higher prevalence of norovirus (Khan, 2009) and even the fungi *Malassezia furfur,* which is naturally found on the skin of humans and other animals and could influence IBD (Limon et al., 2019).

THE CAUSES

The gatekeepers of our colon are the two layers of mucus that line it. IBD is thought to be caused when genetically susceptible individuals are exposed to urban environmental factors that affect their intestinal biomes that lead to thinning of the intestine's mucosa and cause inflammation. In other words, things that compromise the lining of our colon allow pathogens to enter our bloodstream.

Researchers (Chassaing, Koren, Goodrich, Poole, Srinivasan, Ley, & Gewirtz, 2015) found that the ingestion of the emulsifiers carboxymethylcellulose and polysorbate dramatically altered the gut lining by thinning the protective mucus layer.

There are also genetic links to IBD. The first gene linked to Crohn's disease was N0D2. Mutations of N0D2 also have a marked impact on the microbial environment along with the ATG16L1 protein-encoding gene.

The complex genetic-microbe interplay points to several specific factors. Low vitamin D levels as well as having biological relatives with less-diverse intestinal microbiota are both correlated with IBD.

A decrease in some bacteria (*Firmicutes*) and an increase in other bacteria (*Gammaproteobacteria*) have been found by Frank, et al. (2011) and Morgan, et al. (2012) in IBD patients. There are even differences within the same patient when comparing inflamed vs. uninflamed tissue bacterial counts.

A number of studies have also found a relationship between fungi and IBD with more fungal diversity in people with ulcerative colitis and Crohn's disease (Chehoud, et al., 2015; Liguori, et al., 2016 and Sokol, et al., 2017).

Even breastfeeding in infancy seems to lower the risk of developing IBD (Klement, Cohen, Boxman, & Reif, 2004).

IBD has three distinct windows of onset. Early onset IBD occurs at younger than ten years of age. Most IBD occurs between fifteen to thirty years of age, but late onset around age sixty is not uncommon. There is a possibility that the microbiome plays a role in the onset of IBD since developmental changes suspected of affecting the microbiome also occur during these windows.

There is no known singular microbe responsible for IBD; however, a lack of microbial diversity has been observed. Some bacteria (*Enterobacteriaceae*) counts are higher in patients with IBD. As an aside, *Enterobacteriaceae* numbers in strict vegan and vegetarian people are usually lower than in the general population.

Researchers Sartor and Wu (2017) have identified a decrease in protective bacteria like *Bifidobacterium* and an increase in inflammatory microbes like *Protobacteria*, *Fusobacterium* (a bacterium associated with tumor growth) and *E. coli* in patients with IBD.

There is also reason to believe that specific bacteria (sulphate-reducing bacteria) may contribute to IBD, irritable bowel syndrome (IBS), and colorectal cancer.

Many of these bacteria that are important in the production of short chain fatty acids (SCFA) are lacking in the IBD colon. SCFAs are energy sources and nutrition for the colon and are thought to be key components in preventing metabolic syndrome, cancer, ulcerative colitis, and antibiotic-associated diarrhea.

It is important to note that the study of the microbiome is an emerging field. Every day we learn new information. As our knowledge progresses, we may find unique causes for some of the aforementioned correlations about IBD and bacteria. I am always researching new connections and new possibilities. Hope is on the horizon for IBD sufferers.

THE CURES

Treatments for ulcerative colitis and Crohn's have traditionally involved immunosuppressive therapy, mesalamine, glucocorticoids, and tumor necrosis factor antagonists, which rarely cause remission and can significantly diminish the IBD patient's quality of life.

Removal of damaged parts of the colon (colectomy) is too often an undesirable conclusion, but when we consider that IBD is one of the highest risk factors for developing colorectal cancer, efficacious treatments are imperative.

Good news! Like *C. diff*, there is promising evidence that the transplantation of fecal microbiota can lead to remission in ulcerative colitis patients. In a randomized controlled trial, (Borody, Brandt, & Paramsothy, 2003) researchers used FMT to induce remission in ulcerative colitis patients via retention enemas (held in the body for several minutes). Nine of thirty-eight patients achieved remission. The ulcerative colitis patients were eighteen years and older with active UC identified by stool patterns, rectal bleeding, endoscopic findings, and physician assessment. Since retention enemas are not always as efficacious as implantation directly into the cecum, I can only guess that while significant, this success rate could have been much higher. Paramsothy, et al. (2019) conducted another study of ulcerative colitis using FMT and retention enemas and found that remission was associated with Eubacterium and Roseburia species and lack of remission was associated with Fusobacterium, Sutterella, and Escherichia species.

Dr. Faming Zhang and colleagues at the Second Affiliated Hospital of Nanjing Medical University (China)

> **FMT** a.k.a. fecal microbiota transplantation, or **refloralization,** as I like to call it, is the process of transplanting fecal bacteria from a healthy donor into a recipient. FMT involves restoring the colon's microflora by introducing healthy bacterial flora through infusion of stool via colonoscopy, enema, nasogastric tube, or by mouth in the form of a capsule containing stool material from a healthy donor.

recently used FMT to treat fifteen steroid-dependent ulcerative colitis patients. After stopping all medication, patients were given FMT and those who did not respond were given a second FMT. Those who did not respond after the second treatment were then administered a short course of steroid therapy.

Zhang and researchers discovered that 57 percent of the patients showed clinical improvement and discontinued steroid treatment. The gut microbiota of the FMT responders became similar to that of the donor and half of the responders stayed in remission up to eighteen months (Cui et al., 2015).

While the 57 percent response rate is great for those it benefited and those interested in using FMT—it also reinforces the fact that the 43 percent who did not respond may be suffering from a type of ulcerative colitis that may require different therapies.

One way the transplanted microbiota induces remission (healing) is by filling the niches held by pathogens and outcompeting them by taking away their resources. Another way is by boosting T cells, the wrecker service of the bloodstream. T cells get rid of infected or cancerous cells and reduce inflammation. Research by Haden and Gnosh (2008) suggests that microbes influence another mechanism known as NF-κB (nuclear factor kappa-light-chain enhancer of activated B cells), which uses proteins to respond to cellular stress.

A review of fifty-three different FMT studies including forty-one for ulcerative colitis, eleven for Crohn's disease, and four for pouchitis by Paramsothy, et al. (2017) found that overall, 36 percent of ulcerative colitis, 50.5 percent of Crohn's disease, and 21.5 percent of pouchitis (inflamed surgically-created pouch) patients achieved clinical remission. In other words, half of the Crohn's sufferers (forty-three of the eight-five) achieved remission; and more than one-third (201 of 555) of those suffering with ulcerative colitis achieved remission. This means that potentially 244 people could take a salsa dancing class who couldn't do it before! Eat your heart out, Chuck Lorre.

Another study in Australia by Costello, et al. (2019) also found remission rates comparable to previous ones. Twelve of thirty-eight participants with ulcerative colitis went into remission after receiving FMT from a donor. That's another dozen people who could be on the dance floor.

Unfortunately, there is conflicting research by Rossen, et al. (2015) that did not substantiate these remission rates. However, the post-FMT microbiota in the Rossen, et al. study from patients who did respond to FMT had distinct features from that of patients who did not respond to FMT. This evidence also insinuates that maybe there is more than one type of ulcerative colitis or more than one type of dysbiosis. Or possibly, some donor feces are simply better/richer than others. I personally think that using matched donor fecal material yields better results. We would not use A negative blood to infuse someone with a B positive blood type and familial donors usually share many kinds of natural microbiota.

Hopefully optimistic, I think more research may clarify the microbe-gene interaction leading to FMT for the successful treatment of IBD, and because we know that IBD is related to other inflammatory diseases like Lupus and arthritis, there is reason to expect that a whole cluster of diseases may respond to FMT.

While this is an answered prayer for many, I have to wonder about the study's half that didn't respond. Is the reason in the donor bacteria or is it in the diet of the recipient? Is it the genetic bearing of either? Are there unknown pathogens that might need to be addressed?

CHAPTER 7

BE STILL MY HEART

"When you have heart disease, you start to be tired of everything.
It's like getting older. You become more white, and after that, grey.
You have no feeling for anything."
—Gerard Depardieu, French actor

D o you know the number one cause of death in the world? No, it's not bacon—at least not directly. It's heart disease. One in three deaths in the United States is due to heart disease.

All of us have loved someone who died from heart disease. And we are aware of those important numbers we should all know. . . . I'm not talking about your bail bondsman's phone number. I'm talking about the numbers that point to our risk of developing heart

RECIPE FOR A HEART ATTACK:

- Smoke—everything
- Resist activity—sit a lot
- Gain a few lbs.—go big
- Become diabetic
- Amp your cholesterol
- Increase triglycerides
- Lower your HDLs
- Mistake your BP numbers for your IQ

disease: blood pressure, cholesterol, blood glucose (sugar), and body mass. However, recent interest in intestinal inflammation suggests that our microbiome may contribute significantly to these risks. We know that our gut microbes impact our weight. And we know there is evidence that bacteria are a factor in metabolic syndrome, so why wouldn't they affect our heart?

Microbiome research often uses mice that are free of gut flora (germ-free mice). This is important since it is the only way to isolate the effects of the treatment being studied from normal,

> **Arteriosclerosis** a.k.a. **Atherosclerosis** is the thickening and the hardening of arterial walls and the leading cause of heart attacks, stroke, and peripheral vascular disease.

naturally existing microbes. When microbe-free mice are given substances (choline, TMAO, and betaine) known to contribute to heart disease, the dangerous arteriosclerosis-causing metabolites did not form.

In a study of humans treated with broad-spectrum antibiotics, these arteriosclerosis-causing metabolites were markedly lower, but rose after the antibiotics were withdrawn.

Both studies indicate that our bacteria are a factor in the formation of heart disease.

Research by Tang et al. (2015), suggests that increased levels of TMAO (Trimethylamine N-oxide) may be a stronger risk factor for cardiovascular disease than LDLs (low-density lipo-proteins a.k.a. bad choles-terol) and C-reactive proteins

> Trimethylamine N-Oxide or (**TMAO**) is a metabolite manufactured by gut bacteria from lecithin that increases the risk of having a major cardiac event by changing how the body uses cholesterol.

(proteins found in blood whose levels rise in response to inflammation). TMAO is a result of lecithin-rich foods and gut bacteria. Lecithin-rich foods are organ meats, red meats, eggs, seafood, some beans (soybeans, kidney beans, and black beans) and many cooked green vegetables.

> **Lecithin**, from the Greek *lekythos* (egg yolk), is a generic term for yellow-brownish fatty substances occurring in animal and plant tissues, which attract both water and fatty substances. It allows combining two ingredients that do not ordinarily mix easily and repel sticky materials.

Lecithin is an emulsifier that allows two normally opposing ingredients to marry up for all eternity.

Studies suggest that it isn't the food itself that increases the risk of heart disease, but the TMAO produced by the bacteria that breaks down the lecithin in our foods. And our western diet is full of lecithin.

We also know that vegetarians, vegans, and those on the Mediterranean diet are associated with lower TMAO levels and reduced risk for a cardiovascular event.

Research (Yang et al., 2015) in animals with high blood pressure (a risk factor in heart disease) has found dysbiosis in the form of decreased microbial diversity and decreased *Bacteroidetes* to *Firmicutes* ratios.

Collinsella has been found to be increased in patients with atherosclerosis, defined as carotid stenosis when compared to healthy controls who were high in *Roseburia* and *Eubacterium* (Karlsson et al., 2012).

PROBIOTICS

Neither prebiotics nor probiotics have consistently been shown to increase microbial diversity or strengthen bacterial ratios.

Most studies using antibiotics to treat heart disease have been disappointing also. However, new therapies targeting the gut microbiota, including fecal microbiota transplantation, pre/probiotics, and TMAO inhibitors, present new opportunities for the treatment of heart disease (Amadmehrabi and Tang, 2017).

Because of the dietary factors that we know about, looking to FMT or any bacterial treatment may be overreaching until we can identify the entire metabolic pathway that contributes to TMAO. Dietary changes tied to heart disease are a known factor. While controlling TMAO by withholding dietary lecithin is possible, we haven't identified all the bacteria responsible for the lecithin conversion.

CHAPTER 8

OBESITY ETIOLOGY

"If you walk down the street, within five minutes
you will see someone who is morbidly obese or obese."
—**Carnie Wilson, pop singer for Wilson Phillips**

We're a tubby bunch! Since disco died in the 1970s, obesity has tripled. In 2016 the World Health Organization estimated that 39 percent of adults were overweight, and 13 percent were obese. More than ever, people are at risk for cardiovascular disease, diabetes, joint and musculoskeletal disorders, and a number of cancers including breast, ovarian, prostate, liver, gallbladder, kidney, and colon cancers. In the majority of the world, obesity kills more people than starvation. But before you enroll in that salsa dancing class, let's further discuss the role of the intestinal biome in obesity.

With the advent of home computers, more television choices, and cell phones, we have become a group of sedentary consumers. We sit and shop, sit and eat, sit and socialize, and even sit and stare! Between 1988–2009, Chatterjee and DeVol studied the economies and obesity rates in twenty-seven countries. They found that for every 10 percent increase spent on communication and information technology, the obesity rate climbs 1.4 percent. Throw in the internet, and part of our obesity epidemic is a result of global trade agreements that allow more processed foods into the worldwide food supply for corporate profit. Sitting longer, moving less, and eating foods more suited for screen surfing than for health has taken a toll. It has caused worldwide weight woes I call *globesity.*

Researchers have found that an increase of one standard deviation in glo-balization (a multidimensional variable of urbanization, economy, information, technology, etc.) results in a 23 percent increase in obesity and a 4.3 percent increase in caloric intake (Costa-Font & Mas, 2016).

What are processed foods? Foods that have undergone a series of changes (mechanical or chemical) that may also have unhealthy additives. Processed foods are usually frozen, canned, baked, dried, or pasteurized. Examples:

- Bacon
- Bread
- Cereal
- Cheese
- Cookies
- Deli Meats
- Hamburgers
- Hot dogs
- French fries
- Frozen pizza
- Microwave popcorn
- Milk
- Potato chips
- Soft drinks

IMMIGRATION STUDY LINKS WESTERN DIET TO OBESITY

Many processed foods look healthy on the surface, but the problem lies in things like added sugar, fat sodium, preservatives, and emulsifiers. But how does the western diet affect our microbiome? And is our microbiome part of the obesity epidemic?

Vangay, et al. (2018) collected stool from 514 Hmong and Karen hill-tribe individuals living in Thailand and the United States, including first and second-generation immigrants as well as nineteen Karen

Globesity is the effect of mingling worldwide economies and cultures and their effect on obesity and caloric intake.

individuals sampled before and after immigration. Migration from a non-Western country to the United States was associated with immediate loss of gut microbiome diversity. American-associated bacterial strains displaced native strains. These effects increased with duration of US residence and were compounded by obesity.

THE WESTERN DIET DECREASES MICROBIAL DIVERSITY

In 2012, Yatsunenko, et al. found Western human microbiomes to consist of 15 percent to 30 percent fewer species than non-Western microbiomes.

Research in 2017 by Menni, Jackson, Pallister, Steves, Spector, and Valdes found that lower gut microbiome diversity is associated with weight gain. So why do we care about a eubiotic (balanced) microbiome? Because we want airline seats to feel roomy.

In fact, categorizing people as lean or obese can be made solely on the basis of their gut microbiota with 90 percent accuracy (Sun, et al., 2018 and Knights, et al., 2011).

SOME FOOD ADDITIVES THAT ARE NOT ALWAYS OUR FRIENDS:

- Carboxymethylcellulose
- Dextrose
- High-fructose corn syrup
- Hydrogenated oils
- Lecithin
- Nitrates
- Maltose
- Monosodium Glutamate
- Perfluoroalkyls
- Polysorbate
- Trans fats

MICROBIOME CHANGES ARE LINKED TO OTHER RISK FACTORS

A growing body of research suggests that obesity, metabolic syndrome, low-grade inflammation, and insulin resistance are all associated with changes in the intestinal biome (Le Chatelier, et al., 2013). Yes, your swimsuit body may have been kidnapped by the microbiota in your gut.

Research by Cani and Everard (2015) also found increases in specific bacteria in humans and mice on high fat diets. They discovered increases in certain inflammatory molecules (lipopolysaccharides) found on the surface of

> **Metabolic Syndrome** is a group of conditions including high blood pressure, high blood sugar, abdominal fat, and unhealthy cholesterol levels that increase your risk of heart disease, stroke, and diabetes.

bacteria that may cause low grade inflammation, playing a role in insulin resistance, type 2 diabetes, and obesity.

WHAT BACTERIA ARE TO BLAME?

Recent techniques for sequencing microbial DNA have revealed four dominant bacteria types in the gut of mammals (Gram-negative *Bacteroidetes* and *Proteobacteria;* Gram-positive *Actinobacteria* and *Firmicutes*).

Researchers (Ley, Bäckhed, Turnbaugh, Lozupone, Knight, & Gordon, 2005; Turnbaugh, Bäckhed, Fulton, & Gordon, 2008) found that in obese mice, one type of bacteria (*Bacteroidetes*) was reduced and one (*Firmicutes*) was increased when compared to their lean mice siblings on the same diet. They also noted the overall lack of microbiota diversity in obese individuals as well as a reduction in the number of microorganisms.

However, in other research (Arumugam et al., 2011) in which bacteria of thirty-nine people was genetically analyzed—no correlation between body mass index and the Firmicutes/Bacteroidetes ratio was noted. Yet, there were modules (enzymes) on some species that correlated strongly with BMI.

Additional research has found that more exotic microbes rather than the ratios of the dominate ones may be more important in controlling obesity. Research by Zhao, et al. (2019) found that the administration of *Akkermansia muciniphila* bacteria to mice can prevent the development of obesity even though mice probably don't care if their leggings are too tight. However, don't run out and buy *Akkermansia*. There is research that indicates it's a factor in other diseases.

HOW DO GUT BACTERIA MAKE US FAT?

How microbiota influence fat storage and energy extraction is a complicated metabolic process. Researchers (Flint, Scott, Louis, & Duncan, 2012) determined that certain gut microbiota can extract energy from otherwise indigestible starches like the polysaccharides from grains, potatoes, and beans, etc. The gut's microbiome is also able to produce hydrolases (enzymes) that digest carbohydrates into short-chain fatty acids for energy.

Lastly, there are recent writings that explore the interaction between hormones and the microbiome. (Stay tuned for *Let's talk Sh!t 2.0*)

Another way your gut influences your weight is

> **Insulin resistance** is an impaired response of the body to insulin, a hormone that regulates the amount of sugar (glucose) in the blood allowing it to be used for energy. This lack of insulin can lead to type 2 diabetes and is linked to metabolic syndrome and obesity.

its role in **insulin resistance**. Insulin is a hormone made by the pancreas which allows cells to absorb sugar (glucose) so that it can be used as energy. People with insulin resistance are unable to use insulin effectively and this raises sugar levels causing diabetes and its younger sibling: prediabetes. There seems to be a correlation between diabetes and *Proteobacteria.*

Vrieze, et al. (2012) found that the introduction of intestinal microbes from lean donors lead to improvements in insulin levels in patients with metabolic syndrome. Yes, there may be a time when the answer to your weight problem lies in the gut of your svelte sibling.

Leptin is a hormone that tells us when we are full. When rats are given antibiotics (vancomycin), a dramatic decline (38 percent) in circulating leptin levels is observed (Lam, et al., 2012). We can infer that the killing of bacteria is somehow related to the decline in leptin. We also know that when leptin increases in mice, *Mucispirillum, Lactococcus,* and certain *Lachnospiraceae* increases

> ## BY THE NUMBERS
>
> Ideally, adults should aim for these numbers in their health profile:
>
> **Blood pressure** should be from 120 over 80 to less than 140 over 90.
>
> **Blood sugar** levels should be less than 100 mg/dL after not eating for at least eight hours. Less than 140 mg/dL two hours after eating.
>
> **Body mass index** is now used in lieu of weight. A BMI of:
> - Under 18.5 is underweight
> - 18.5 to 24.9 is healthy
> - 25.0 to 29.9 is usually unhealthy
>
> **LDL cholesterol** should be less than 100 mg/dl. Over 189 mg/dL is very high.
>
> **HDL cholesterol** should be between 40 milligrams per deciliter and 60 milligrams per deciliter.

(Ravussin, et al., 2012) and other bacteria like *Allobaculum* are negatively correlated with leptin levels.

Ghrelin stimulates appetite, increases food intake, and promotes fat storage. Ghrelin is negatively correlated with the abundance of *Bifidobacterium, Lactobacillus* and *B. coccoides*, and positively correlated with a number of *Bacteroides* and *Prevotella* species (Queipo-Ortuno, et al., 2013).

All of this could mean that when your skinny brother or your slim sister eats the same food that causes you to gain weight, it is up to the bacteria running the food distillation system in the gut that determines how much of those nachos goes to fat and how much of them produces energy. Before you call your svelte sibling up and plead your "It's not my fault!" case—keep reading. *It gets better.*

Body Mass Index or **BMI** is our weight in kilograms divided by our height in meters squared between 25.0 and 29.9 kg/m², and an obese person as someone with a BMI greater or equal to 30.0 kg/m². However, BMI can't distinguish between fat and muscle (which tends to be heavier) and can put more muscular individuals into overweight status, even if their fat levels are low.

Weight loss is at the forefront of almost everyone's to do list. It is the topmost New Year's resolution and comes up in conversations at an alarming rate. We want *skinny*. We want to be able to shop for swimwear without becoming nauseated.

We also want the luxury of buying all the foods, all the time. This means that much of our food comes from global markets when they are out of season at local growers. They may harbor microbes, so bacteria you hadn't had contact with a few decades ago are now on a grocer's shelf near you.

For example, during our Northern Hemisphere winter, Southern Hemisphere countries like Chile, Argentina, and South Africa are selling us their summertime grapes while Southern California is shipping strawberries to Japan.

In the past, our natural human microbiomes were tailored to our local and culturally traditional food supply. Now, we ship foods all over the planet, resulting in a world-wide microbiome shift. Is this good or bad? If we know that decreasing microbial diversity is linked to obesity, it could be good. But we also know that the introduction of new bacteria can come with costs. There may be bacteria introduced in our food chain that our own microbiome is not accustomed to that causes dysbiosis. These are questions that can only be answered by research and time.

MORE FOOD FOR THOUGHT

Taking oligofructose (a prebiotic that promotes growth of *Bifidobacterium* and *Lactobacillus*) decreases secretion of ghrelin in obese humans according to Parnell and Reimer (2009). However, the idea that there is a miracle cure for $19.95 (or any price) that will solve our weight problem is rarely true. Because we live in a marketing-driven society, there is no end to the so-called *solutions* that can be purchased. Pills, equipment, supplements, lotions, and potions—all promising that our dreams can come true.

My advice: be a skeptical consumer. What helps one person may not fix another. It is this uniqueness that makes us a small, but important part of the global biome. Don't be persuaded by commercials for miracles. Consider your own environment, habits, DNA, and maybe even your unique microbiota.

I have come to appreciate what we *don't* know. The knowledge we have yet to discover is far greater than what we have found thus far. Even as I write this, I understand that knowledge is being obtained at an incredible rate. What I write today may not be relevant tomorrow. But the pathway to understanding is not a straight line but a road of curves and dead ends. Ask questions, dare to disagree.

THE POSSIBILITIES

All of these findings suggest that FMT from lean donors—perhaps, your thin siblings—could lead to a healthier, leaner you. So, when you make that phone call, remember—one day you might be asking a lot of your brother or sister. Proceed with caution, even if your birthday is coming up. And don't get your hopes too high. A recent study at Brigham and Women's Hospital found that FMT capsules (from a lean donor) were safe but did not reduce BMI. However, the FMT capsules were well tolerated and led to changes in the intestinal microbiome and bile acid profiles that were similar to those of the lean donor (Allegretti, et al., 2019).

Research published in 2019 (Scheiman, et al.) discovered that the gut bacteria *Veillonella* found in elite athletes may play a role in boosting their performance. Researchers isolated a strain of *Veillonella* from a marathon runner and inserted it into the colons of lab mice, and found that the mice given *Veillonella* were able to run 13 percent longer on a treadmill compared to mice who were not given the bacteria. However promising this research may be, do not go out and buy *Veillonella* to improve your BMI! Much more research is needed before QVC should sell designer *Veillonella*.

CHAPTER 9

ON LYME

"As a general rule, the longer the Lyme has been present,
the longer the antibiotic treatment will last."
—Kenneth Singleton, *The Lyme Disease Solution*

A cluster of afflictions thought to be juvenile rheumatoid arthritis was identified in the mid-1970s in the town of Old Lyme, Connecticut. In 1981, a bacterium was described by American scientist Wilhelm (Willy) Burgdorfer (1925–2014) as the cause. The bacterium became known as *Borrelia burgdorferi* and is transmitted to humans through the bite of infected ticks. *B. burgdorferi* has never been identified as part of a healthy human microbiome and as of this writing is always considered a pathogen.

Every year the CDC can easily confirm thirty thousand cases of Lyme disease, but there is reason to believe another 270,000 cases or more may exist and simply be underreported. The number of US counties affected by Lyme disease has increased 320 percent in the past twenty years (Kugeler, et al., 2011). Lyme disease was traditionally more prevalent in the Northeast but now has been found in all fifty states and the District of Columbia, according to Quest Diagnostics. Lyme's wide

Lyme disease rash: The first sign of infection is usually a circular or "bull's-eye" rash called **erythema migrans** or EM, which occurs in approximately 70–80 percent of those infected and begins at the site of a tick bite.

range of symptoms can occur anywhere from three to thirty days after the bite. In some cases, symptoms can appear months after the bite and can mimic those of several ailments, making it difficult to diagnose.

The critter usually responsible for Lyme disease is the black-legged tick and it must be attached to you for thirty-six to forty-eight hours to transmit the disease-causing bacteria. If you remove the tick within forty-eight hours, you are unlikely to get infected.

ANTIBIOTICS ARE TRADITIONALLY THE FIRST LINE OF DEFENSE

According to the CDC, Lyme disease can be treated successfully by antibiotics if caught within a few weeks using doxycycline, amoxicillin, or cefuroxime axetil.

However, if Lyme disease is left untreated, the infection can spread to joints, the heart, and the nervous system. About 10 percent of people treated for Lyme disease will continue to have symptoms. Those people usually have joint or muscle

Antimicrobials are a class of drugs that includes antibiotics, antifungals, antiprotozoals, and antivirals. Antibiotics are produced naturally from molds or bacteria.

Antimicrobials can be synthesized, but the term encompasses both.

pain, fatigue, and short-term memory loss or mental confusion. This has been called post-treatment Lyme disease syndrome, but because the symptoms are common to many inflammatory illnesses the diagnosis is not widely accepted.

Using antibiotics to treat Lyme or any infection is a prime example of antimicrobial medicine—and it was discovered by accident.

Scientists had known for years that Egyptians were known to treat wounds with moldy bread, but it wasn't until 1922, while infected with a cold, that Scottish

> ## SYMPTOMS OF LYME DISEASE MAY INCLUDE THE FOLLOWING:
>
> **Flu-like symptoms that come and go:**
> - Achy, stiff, swollen joints
> - Anxiety
> - Dizziness
> - Ear ringing
> - Fatigue
> - Fever
> - Headaches
> - Jaw pain
> - Mood swings
> - Neck pain
> - Night sweats
> - Rashes
> - Trouble sleeping
>
> **Heart problems:**
> - Chest pain
> - Palpitations
> - Shortness of breath
>
> **Neurological symptoms:**
> - Concentration problems
> - Light sensitivity
> - Loss of taste or smell
> - Skin tingling, numbness
> - Weakness or paralysis of face

physician-scientist Alexander Fleming accidently sneezed on a Petri dish. Not known for his laboratory organization, Fleming set the dish on his cluttered desk and left it. Two weeks later he found that numerous colonies of bacteria had grown, but the area where the mucus had been remained clear. The mucous had its own antibacterial powers. In 1928, Fleming launched experiments involving the common staphylococcal bacteria. An uncovered Petri dish sitting next to an open window began accidentally growing mold. (He probably could've used a good lab assistant.) Fleming found that the bacteria close to the mold colony were dying. He was able to isolate the mold and identified it as a member of

> **Lyme neuroborreliosis** is a type of neurological Lyme disease, caused by a systemic infection of spirochetes of the genus *Borrelia*. Symptoms include spinal pain in the lumbar and cervical regions, radiating to the extremities, cranial nerve abnormalities, and altered mental faculties. Sensory findings may also be present. Rarely, a progressive form of encephalomyelitis may occur.

the *Penicillium* genus. He found it to be effective against bacteria that caused diseases such as scarlet fever, pneumonia, gonorrhea, meningitis, and diphtheria. He decided that it was not the mold itself but some sort of juice the mold had produced that had killed the bacteria. He named this moldy juice, "penicillin."

He was later quoted as saying, "When I woke up just after dawn on September 28, 1928, I certainly didn't plan to revolutionize all medicine by discovering the world's first antibiotic, or bacteria killer. But I suppose that was exactly what I did."

It wasn't until 1940 that two other scientists, Howard Florey and Ernst Chain, figured out how to use penicillin as a drug. It took two thousand liters of mold juice to obtain enough penicillin to treat a single case of human sepsis. But in 1941, lab assistant Mary Hunt offered up a couple of over-ripe melons covered in a robust golden mold and the lab went ballistic.

The mold turned out to be *Penicillium chrysogeum*, which yielded two hundred times the amount of penicillin that Fleming described. After mutation-causing X-rays and filtration, the genetically modified fungus yielded one thousand times as much penicillin as its fungal antecedents.

In 1945, Fleming, Florey, and Chain were awarded the Nobel Prize. In Fleming's acceptance speech, he warned that the overuse of penicillin could cause bacterial resistance. And what of Mary Hunt? She wasn't recognized. I'm just hoping that you'll remember this story when you become a *Jeopardy* finalist.

Here in the twenty-first century, we still don't completely understand this delicate microorganism dance that cures some and condemns others. Antibiotics do work for many people with Lyme disease, but for others there is a lifetime of challenges.

Researchers think that imbalances in the microbiome from Lyme disease create inflammation by stimulating metabolic pathways (cytokines) that result in inflammation (Pachner & Steiner, 2007; Lochhead, et al., 2017; Soloski, Crowder, Lahey, Wagner, Robinson, & Aucott, 2014). These inflammatory responses are responsible for some of the symptoms seen in Lyme disease, especially those with what is called *post-treatment Lyme disease syndrome*. This syndrome includes antibiotic-resistant arthritis after treatment and has led to wide speculation as to cause, but it is still not fully understood.

As a doctor, I understand that bacteria like *Borrelia burgdorferi* needs to be restrained, and I understand that antibiotics work. But maybe they work too well and play a role in the persistence of arthritis after the initial infection. Is it possible to cure post-treatment Lyme disease with richer, more diverse microorganisms? Perhaps.

All of this leads us to question the relationship between antibiotics and inflammation, and then the natural follow-up question about the relationship between inflammation and the microbiome. Should a bacterial infection be treated with its natural bacterial enemies? Is it more complex than simply wiping out the infecting bacteria, a.k.a. pathogens? Is our human microbiome the equivalent to a black hole in the universe? So vast and so dense that we might never truly understand it.

Chapter 10

SPECTRUM SPECULATION

"We cry, we scream, we hit . . . and break things. But still, we don't
want you to give up on us. Please, keep battling alongside us."
—Naoki Higashida, autism sufferer

Autism, bacteria, and therapy are three words we never thought
would be linked—until recently. Autism is defined as a disorder
of variable severity whose hallmark resides in difficulty with social interaction, communication, and repetitive thoughts and behaviors.

Some autism sufferers have intellectual disabilities with lower intelligence quotients (IQs). However, many have above average intelligence.
It is becoming more accepted that autism has nothing to do with intelligence. Communication challenges simply make the autistic more difficult test subjects.

Diagnoses of autism have sky-rocketed in recent years—up 15 percent in two years. One in fifty-nine children are diagnosed with autism
spectrum disorder (ASD). Estimates claim it may be as high as one in
thirty-eight among boys.

The first documented case of autism goes back to a 1747 court case
where the brother of Hugh Blair of Borgue in Scotland petitioned to annul

Blair's marriage to his wife, hoping to get Blair's inheritance. Court documents describe Blair as exhibiting strong autistic symptoms.

In 1798, a feral child in France named Victor of Aveyron who'd lived in the wild for several years was brought back into society. He became known as The Wild Boy of Aveyron. A young medical student, Jean

> ## COMMON REPETITIVE AUTISTIC BEHAVIORS:
> * Flipping levers
> * Hand flapping
> * Head-banging
> * Lining up toys
> * Opening and closing drawers or doors
> * Rocking
> * Shaking sticks
> * Spinning

Marc Gaspard Itard, effectively adopted Victor into his home and tried to educate him. Extensive documentation was taken as Itard attempted to teach the boy language and social skills. It is thought that Victor most likely suffered from autism.

Then in 1911, a psychiatrist from Switzerland, Eugen Bleuler, used the term autism to describe a unique cluster of symptoms that were originally thought to be schizophrenia. Since then, scientific research approached the causes of autism with many vigorous, diverse hypotheses. Possible causes have included genetic predisposition, measles in the pregnant mother, lack of oxygen at birth, environmental chemicals, vaccines, and viruses—among many others. Parents have even blamed circumcision! Because autistic behaviors are rarely seen before a year of age, parents are quick to take note of changes in their child's behavior and look to recent events for cause.

Brain scans of autistic children have revealed differences in the shapes and structures when compared to their non-autistic counterparts (Sato et al., 2017 and Erbetta, et al., 2014). However, other research found brain differences

People with **Asperger Syndrome** share many of the same social interaction challenges as those with autism. However, there is no developmental delay of speech. They are usually average or above in intelligence, but may have an obsessive focus on a certain topic or perform the same behaviors again and again.

in the non-autistic parents of their autistic children who exhibited the same brain characteristics as other autistic children (Rojas, Smith, Benkers, Camou, Reite, & Rogers, 2004).

In 2013, the term autism was changed to autism spectrum disorder (ASD) and now includes other disorders like Asperger Syndrome and Pervasive Developmental Disorder Not Otherwise Specified.

ANOTHER APPROACH

We know that gastrointestinal issues can lead to behavioral changes in mice (remember *Ratatouille*?), but research by Lyte, Varcoe, and Bailey (1998) found that *Campylobacter jejuni*, the bacteria that causes food poisoning, decreased exploratory behavior and increased nonexploratory behaviors in mice.

Other researchers (Castex, Fioramonti, de Lahitte, Luffau, More, & Bueno, 1998) discovered that the bacteria *Nippostrongylus*, a roundworm or nematode that infects rodents, activated pulmonary and intestinal inflammation which is associated with motor disorders.

Lyte, Li, Opitz, Gaykema, and Goehler (2006) noticed increased anxiety in mice after the administration of the bacteria *Citrobacter rodentium*. *Citrobacter rodentium* is a mouse pathogen that mimics human *Escherichia coli* and causes acute colitis. This was not your typical Disney adventure. It was a springboard for the investigation of the relationship between nerves that connect the gut and the brain and the link between behavior and bacteria.

After which, more researchers (Goehler, Park, Opitz, Lyte, & Gaykema, 2007) found that the bacteria *Campylobacter jejuni*, a common cause of food poisoning, increases anxiety-like behavior in mice.

This connection logically suggests that some neuropsychiatric disorders may be due to dysbiosis. Other studies have found a link between depression and bacteria. While we think of depression as originating in our brain, the gut-brain axis is linked by bacteria. And when we look at the connection between IBD and depression, it makes sense that the behavioral aspects of depression could be influenced by bacteria.

A recent study in Belgium found the bacteria, *Coprococcus* and *Dialister* missing from the microbiomes of the depressed subjects but not from those subjects with a high quality of life (Valles-Colomer et al., 2019).

Another study (Finegold, Summanen, Downes, Corbett, & Komoriya, 2017) published in *Anaerobe* found that the microbiome of thirty-three autistic children was colonized by higher numbers of *Clostridium perfringens*, a bacterium thought to produce toxins.

In 2017, Arizona State University confirmed lower overall microbial diversity and reduced relatives of the *Prevotella copri* bacteria in children with ASD. Lower numbers of *Feacalibacterium prausnitzii* and Haemophilus parainfluenzae were also found in children with ASD (Kang et al., 2017). Kang and the gang kept researching and in 2019 they followed up on eighteen subjects with ASD that had been treated with "modified-FMT trial with an intensive combination called Microbial Transfer Therapy (MTT) consisting of two-week vancomycin treatment followed by a bowel cleanse and then high dose FMT for one to two days and seven to eight weeks of daily maintenance doses along with a stomach-acid suppressant, administered to children with

ASD and chronic gastrointestinal problems." Eight weeks after the end of the treatment, they found an 80 percent reduction in GI symptoms and a slow-but-steady improvement in ASD symptoms. They also found that gut microbial diversity, including potentially beneficial microbes, had significantly increased.

Two years later, they followed up on the original eighteen ASD subjects and discovered something amazing. The families reported that ASD-related symptoms had slowly, steadily improved since week eighteen. The parents used a Social Responsiveness Scale (SRS) revealing that 89 percent of the ASD subjects were in the severe range at the beginning of the trial, but the percentile dropped to 47 percent at the two-year follow-up. Other parent-completed scales, as well as those by professional evaluators, also indicated improvement.

Since *Bifidobacterium* and *Prevotella* remained higher in the feces of participants at the two-year follow-up, the researchers concluded that ASD behavior and GI symptoms were significantly correlated (Kang et al., 2019).

These encouraging observations demonstrate that the intensive MTT intervention is a promising therapy for treating children with ASD who have GI problems.

While FMT might not cure autism, it could change the course of the disease. Changing behavioral symptoms, and improving the quality of life might be a huge step for autism sufferers and their families and friends.

CHAPTER 11

EPIDERMAL DETERRENT

"Your skin is really a great indicator of what's going on inside your body."
—Sami Blackford, holistic skincare specialist

I f there's anything that will keep us home on Friday night, it's ugly, unhealthy skin. There are many things we can move past, but if we have raw oozing sores, our self-esteem goes into free fall. No one wants to kiss someone with a cold sore or hug someone with hives.

By now, it should be no surprise that researchers have found a connection between our microbiome and the health of our skin. Smeekens, et al. (2014) linked people with a **primary immunodeficiency disease (PIDD)** to differences in their microbiome using oral and skin microbial counts. They discovered that people with **chronic mucocutaneous candidiasis a.k.a. CMC** (a group of inherited disorders characterized by recurrent infections of the skin, nails, and mucus membranes due to the pathogen *Candida albicans)* and those with **hyper IgE** syndrome had more *Acinetobacter* bacteria and less *Corynebacterium* compared to their healthy counterparts.

Both of these genetic diseases increase the risk of fungal and *Staphylococcus* infections.

PIDD is a group of over three hundred chronic diseases caused by a weak immune system thought to be genetic in origin and usually diagnosed in childhood. Symptoms can be severe and/or reoccurring and may include pneumonia, sinus infections, abscesses, ear infections, and skin infections to name a few.

Examples of PIDD:

- Agammaglobulinemia
- Ataxia-telangectasia
- BENTA Disease
- Chronic granulomatous
- CTLA$_4$ Deficiency
- DiGeorge syndrome
- DOCK$_8$ Deficiency
- GATA$_2$ Deficiency
- Wiscott-Aldrich syndrome
- Selective IgA deficiency

Another chronic skin condition, psoriasis vulgaris, has also been linked to the microbiome. A hundred million people worldwide suffer from this disease, but it was Cindi Lauper's battle with psoriasis that made this once unheard-of disease far more recognizable. Psoriasis is thought to be caused by an overactive immune system, which speeds up the life cycle of skin cells. Symptoms include redness, flaking, thickening patches of skin (plaques) that may be white, silver, or red in color, along with dry-cracked skin that may bleed. It's accompanied by itching, burning, or soreness.

It does not turn one's hair pink, though. That is a whole different can of germs.

Psoriasis symptoms are usually different for everyone, and some people will experience joint swelling and stiffness. Most psoriasis sufferers have periods of remission interrupted by weeks or months of flares.

Psoriasis has tradition-
ally been treated with corti-
costeroid creams, retinoids
(vitamin A ointments), sal-
icylic acid ointments, cal-
citriol (synthetic vitamin
D3) ointment, and coal-tar
ointments as well as photo-

> **Hyper IgE Syndrome** is a
> rare immunodeficiency disease
> characterized by eczema,
> eosinophilia, skin abscesses, lung
> infections, and high serum levels
> of **IgE**.

therapy (light therapy), methotrexate (cancer chemotherapy), oral retinoids, and biologics.

While psoriasis is often thought of as a skin disorder, there is reason
to believe that it is part of a systemic inflammatory disease involving
both skin and gut microbiomes. Arthritis and inflammatory bowel disease are also associated with spondyloarthritis. Only until recently has
the complicated relationship between different inflammatory diseases
and microbes been explored.

Psoriasis, like many diseases, is thought to be a combination of
genetics and environmental factors (Merve, et al., 2017). However, a
substantial body of research has found that dysbiosis of the gut and skin
microbiome is associated with psoriasis (Cohen, Dreiher, & Birkenfeld,
2009; Goa, Tseng, Strober, Pei, & Blaser, 2008; Eppinga, Konstantinov,
Peppelenbosch, & Thio, 2014; H Tett et al., 2017; Codoñer et al., 2018).

People with psoriasis
have been found to have
decreased *Bacteroidetes* and
increased *Faecalibacteria*
in their gut microbiome.
They also have been found
to have less microbial diversity (Scher et al., 2015).

> What are biologics? **Biologics**
> are drugs made from human
> and animal proteins. They block
> enzymes that cause inflammation.
> Biologics are effective but
> expensive.

> **Spondyloarthritis** is a group of inflammatory diseases that involves both the joints and the entheses (the sites where the ligaments and tendons attach to the bones). It includes **ankylosing spondylitis** and **psoriatic arthritis**. Common symptoms are joint pain sometimes affecting the spine.

Psoriasis sufferers also tend to have more *Staphylococcus* and *Streptococcus* on their skin. Codoñer, et al. (2018) found a core microbiome (enterotype) in psoriasis vulgaris sufferers that differs from those in healthy individuals.

There is hope! A Danish research team (Kragsnaes, et al., 2017) is conducting FMTs on eighty patients with psoriatic arthritis. For a complete read of their research, Google: Efficacy and safety of fecal microbiota transplantation in patients with psoriatic arthritis: protocol for a six-month, double-blind, randomized, placebo-controlled trial.

CHAPTER 12

INFLAMMATION RATIONALIZATION

"The immune system triggers inflammation when the body is confronted with a potential threat, like a harmful chemical or microbe. That process can become problematic when inflammation becomes the body's default state. And evidence suggests that conditions from Alzheimer's to depression, cancer, and heart disease, could be caused by chronic inflammation."
—Newsweek

What is inflammation? It's a word we're familiar with. If we get a cut or a bruise, we can see the redness and swelling that invades the damaged skin. Ouch! This is inflammation we can see and feel. But what about the kind of inflammation that we can't see? The kind that is linked to arthritis, heart disease, and inflammatory bowel disease.

There are at least eighteen different kinds of inflammation. However, the one associated with our microbiome is **chronic inflammation** lasting for months to years. Worldwide, three out of five deaths are from chronic inflammatory diseases like chronic respiratory diseases, heart disorders, cancers, obesity, and diabetes.

WHAT CAUSES CHRONIC INFLAMMATION?

Like autism, chronic inflammation has been blamed on numerous causes. Because the metabolic pathways that lead to inflammation are complicated, I will try to simplify this without resorting to specifics: enzymes, proteins, cytokines, genes, macrophages, and lymphocytes that contain more acronyms, numbers, and explanations than a teenager texting.

Chronic inflammation can be a result of **infectious bacteria, viruses, and fungi**. Illnesses like tuberculosis, Lyme disease, and *C. diff* have been linked to specific bacteria.

> ### RISK FACTORS FOR CHRONIC INFLAMMATION:
> - Age—chance of chronic inflammation increases with age
> - Diet—high amounts of saturated fat, trans-fats, or refined sugar
> - Hormones—low estrogen and testosterone
> - Obesity—BMI is related to cytokine release
> - Sleep disorders
> - Smoking—lowers anti-inflammatory molecules
> - Stress—increases cytokine release

Researchers suspect that liver disease, type 2 diabetes, Parkinson's, and Alzheimer's diseases may also be linked to ill-behaved bacteria (Wassenaar and Zimmermann, 2018). However, these diseases are not active infections, but are caused by normally dormant bacteria that have been stressed and begin to replicate and secrete lipopolysaccharides (LPS), which are inflammatory-driving toxins that come from within. **Irritants** can also cause chronic inflammation. I'm not referring to telemarketers, but industrial irritants like asbestos or everyday allergies to fur, dander, and pollen, which can irritate lungs. Asbestos exposure accounts for 3–4 percent of all lung cancers. Some studies have found that talcum powder that contains asbestos has also been linked to chronic inflammation.

Too much smoke from any source causes lung inflammation, increasing C-reactive proteins (made by the liver in response to inflammation) and white blood cell counts (systemic indicators

TYPES OF INFLAMMATION:

- acute
- catarrhal
- chronic
- exudative
- fibrinous
- granulomatous
- hyperplastic
- interstitial
- parenchymatous
- plastic
- productive
- proliferous
- pseudomembranous
- purulent
- serous
- subacute
- suppurative
- ulcerative

of inflammation) leading to COPD, emphysema, and an increased risk for lung cancer.

Autoimmune disorders cause chronic inflammation. Autoimmune diseases are caused when the immune system mistakenly attacks the body's own healthy tissue and are thought to be the result of genetics, environment, and lifestyle. Rheumatoid arthritis, systemic lupus, celiac disease, PIDD, and multiple sclerosis are examples of autoimmune diseases that can lead to chronic inflammation.

Obesity is linked to some diagnostic markers for inflammation. Obese people are at higher risk for heart disease, cancer, and diabetes. Fat cells can trigger the release of cytokines, but instead of attacking an invader, they go after healthy nerves, organs, or

Cytokines are various proteins secreted by different cells that manage the immune system. Cytokines target immune cells and bind with receptors on them. The binding triggers immune cells. Too much triggering can cause inflammation.

tissues. More weight gain leads to more of these cytokines, affecting our body's ability to use insulin, sometimes leading to type 2 diabetes.

WHAT HAPPENS IN THE INFLAMMATORY PROCESS?

All inflammatory processes start the same. Blood vessels dilate to increase blood flow, then capillaries open to allow neutrophils (white blood cells) access to the afflicted tissue. The white blood cells become macrophages and lymphocytes that replace the neutrophils. However, chronic inflammation continues to produce macrophages, lymphocytes, and plasma cells that make inflammatory cytokines, growth factors, and enzymes that contribute to tissue damage. It's a lot

> ## SIGNS OF CHRONIC INFLAMMATION:
> - Aches and pains
> - Depression and mood swings
> - Excess mucus production
> - Fatigue and insomnia
> - Frequent infections
> - Gastrointestinal problems:
>   - Constipation
>   - Diarrhea
>   - Acid reflux
> - Skin rashes
> - Weight gain or loss

like having two dozen well-intentioned friends who offer to help paint your house. Before long they are stepping all over each other: some walls will get painted twice, some will get the wrong color, and some will be missed completely. Someone will bring beer, there will be mistakes.

HOW DOES OUR MICROBIOME FIT IN?

In 2013, researchers linked low microbial diversity to intestinal inflammation, obesity, insulin resistance, and low-grade inflammation (Le Chatlier, et al., 2013). Since then, a number of studies have linked dysbiosis and inflammation (Sartor, 2014; Cenit, Olivares, Codoñer-Franch, & Sanz, 2015; Jiang, Wu, Wang, Chi, Zhang et al., 2015).

Microbes in the intestine have also been known to alter cancer risk when responding to inflammation by increasing cell proliferation. They can often limit or facilitate tumor growth (Cho & Blaser, 2012; Plottel & Blaser, 2011). People infected with *H. pylori* have increased inflammatory cytokine function (protein messengers) that increases gastric acids (Noach, Rolf, & Tytgat et al, 1994) which can cause ulcers and stomach cancer. However, *H. pylori* in the esophagus and airways can prevent disease. This is one of those situations where everyone needs to stay in their own lane.

When Zhao, et al. (2016) fed mice *A. muciniphilia,* it reduced inflammation and allowed them to lose weight. This doesn't mean you should start *A. muciniphilia* therapy. As I've noted in previous chapters, bacterium can be good or bad, depending on its balance with other bacteria or its location.

ONE PIECE OF THE PUZZLE

Leptin levels increase during inflammation (Mancuso, et al., 2002; Moshyedi, et al., 1998; Sarraf, et al., 1997). Leptin is the hormone that tells our brain (hypothalamus) when we are full. Several studies have suggested that leptin in the intestine epithelium may play a part against gut pathogens and play a role in shaping the microbiome (Rajala et al., 2014).

Leptin-deficient mammals develop obesity. If this is true, why is weight gain a symptom of chronic inflammation? Why wouldn't all that leptin just slim us down like it does our lab rat counterparts?

Because metabolic pathways are complicated journeys, researchers are looking at things like **leptin resistance**. It could be because of the chronic inflammation and tiredness that you are not expending energy, which is another part of the leptin feedback loop. Leptin can reduce the number of calories you burn. Since leptin resistance is a newcomer to metabolism, many researchers and doctors can't even agree on a definition. So, while we know it may be a player in the microbiome, its exact role is unknown.

INFLAMMATORY DISEASES

Celiac disease starts with genetic susceptibility. Celiac genes are present in 30–40 percent of the general population but only about one percent of the population is diagnosed with celiac. Gluten (a protein in grains including wheat, barley, and rye) is the environmental trigger for celiac causing inflammation in the small intestinal mucosa.

However, gluten does not trigger everyone with the celiac genes and some people are diagnosed as adults after

Immunosuppressive drugs are used to suppress various autoimmune conditions. They are usually divided into several categories:

Glucocorticoids are used to treat arthritis, lupus, Crohn's, eczema, and allergies among other autoimmune disorders. Cortisone and prednisone are examples of glucocorticoids.

Cytostatics like methotrexate inhibit cell division and are used for rheumatoid arthritis and lupus.

Antibody drugs are used for autoimmune and cancer treatment. Drugs acting on **immunophilins** are used mainly as anti-rejection drugs after transplants.

TNF binding protein drugs are used in the treatment of psoriasis, rheumatoid arthritis, ankylosing spondylitis, and Crohn's disease. These drugs may raise the risk of contracting tuberculosis.

many years of gluten consumption (Sanz, 2015). It is thought that viral or bacterial infections may somehow trigger gluten intolerance in these people, perhaps by changing their intestinal microbes.

Several studies have found microbiota counts in celiac sufferers that are distinct from their healthy counterparts even after maintaining a gluten-free diet. Celiac patients have increased *Bacteroides* and *Proteobacteria* (Collado, Donat, Ribes-Koninckx, Calabuig, & Sanz, 2008; Schippa, et al., 2010). Celiac patients also have higher numbers of *Staphylococcus* (Collado, Calabuig, & Sanz, 2007; Di Cagno, et al., 2009). However, they also have fewer *Bifidobacterium* (Collado, et al., 2009; Di Cagno, et al., 2009 and 2011). These findings are still under scrutiny while researchers (like ourselves) continue genetic sequencing.

Psoriatic arthritis (PsA) is an autoimmune disease of the skin and joints with bacterial associations (Eppinga et al., 2014; Coit & Sawalha, 2016; Ciccia, et al., 2016). Psoriatic arthritis is a type of inflammatory arthritis that affects some psoriasis sufferers. Most develop psoriasis first and are later diagnosed with psoriatic arthritis, but joint problems sometimes begin before the skin lesions appear.

Several intestinal bacteria including *Akkermansia* and *Ruminococcus* are lacking in patients with PsA. These bacteria are not only important for gut homeostasis, but throwing their names around will impress the relatives. Research is ongoing that may shed light on the possibility of treating psoriatic arthritis (Kragsnaes, et al., 2017) with bacterial products.

Different types of arthritis are linked to specific bacterial dysbiosis. **Rheumatoid arthritis** (RA) is an autoimmune disease in which the body's immune system mistakenly attacks the joints. This creates inflammation that causes the lining inside of joints (the synovium) to thicken, resulting in joint swelling and pain. Sufferers may have firm lumps under the skin in joint areas. Researchers (Scher, et al., 2013) found increases in *Prevotella copri* and decreases in *Bacteroides* in new-onset untreated rheumatoid arthritis patients. This is an area of study that needs more research for verification.

Spondyloarthritis (SpA) is a group of inflammatory diseases that involve the joints and the sites where the ligaments and tendons attach to the bones. Increases in *Ruminicoccus gnavus* bacterium have been found in the feces of SpA patients when compared to healthy controls (Breban, et al., 2017). Again, much more data needs to be collected on SpA and *R. gnavus* before any conclusions can be drawn.

Osteoarthritis is the most common type of arthritis and occurs when the cartilage on the ends of your bones wears down over time. It was traditionally thought of as non-inflammatory but has recently been revisited as having inflammatory sub-types. Links between the microbiome and bone health have not been well studied. However, changes in the gut microbiota have been associated with many of the factors that cause osteoporosis and fractures.

An absence of microbiota has been associated with altered bone mass in mice (Sjögren, et al., 2012). Estrogen depletion alone does not result in bone loss in germ-free mice (Li, et al., 2016), and probiotics can sometimes prevent bone loss. Inflammatory bowel disease is related to the microbiome and is known to lead to osteopenia, a weakening of the bones, (Ali, Lam, Bronze, & Humphrey, et al., 2009).

Patients with inflammatory bowel disease are at higher risk of developing osteoporosis and osteopenia than the general population. The risk of fracture is 40 percent higher in patients with inflammatory bowel disease (Compston, et al., 1987).

Asthma and allergies are also inflammatory illnesses that are believed to be associated with the microbiome. Allergic diseases have steadily increased over the last few decades. Once thought of as sterile, the lungs seem to be a microbiome all their own. The discovery of various bacteria phyla, including *Actinobacteria, Bacteroidetes, Firmicutes,* and *Proteobacteria* has been found in healthy subjects. It is possible that the gut and lung mucosa may function as one organ that shares immunological functions (Segal, et al., 2014).

Depression studies point to a finding that the same microbes responsible for gut inflammation may also be responsible for depression.

Research at Peking University in Beijing found that patients with IBS, diarrhea, and depression have similar alterations in fecal microbiota (Liu, et al., 2016). The fecal samples in the depressed IBS group were less diverse than those in the healthy control group. But, wouldn't anyone with IBS and diarrhea be depressed? And if they weren't depressed, wouldn't you wonder why?

Well, scientists have found that you can just slap someone out of it. Researchers at the University of Southend in the UK slapped over a thousand people and found that 75 percent of them reported improvement in depression symptoms. NO! I made that up. You have to be a skeptic. There is no University of Southend in the UK. Southend is one of a few major cities in the UK without a university. However, if

SYMPTOMS OF DEPRESSION:

- Trouble concentrating
- Can't recall details
- Difficulty with decisions
- Tiredness
- Feelings of:
  - guilt
  - worthlessness
  - helplessness
  - pessimism
  - hopelessness
- Sleep problems:
  - insomnia
  - waking too early
  - sleeping too much
  - restlessness
- Irritability
- Loss of interest in things that were once pleasurable:
  - sex
  - hobbies
  - exercise
- Overeating or loss appetite
- Aches and pains
- Digestive problems that don't get better with treatment
- Suicidal thoughts

there were a University of Southend, they probably could do some very serious fecal research. Always question the data!

A research paper in *Nature Microbiology* titled, "The neuroactive potential of the human gut microbiota in quality of life and depression," found specific groups of microorganisms that positively or negatively correlated with mental health. A team of Belgium researchers (Valles-Collomer, et al., 2019) found that some species of *Coprococcus* and *Dialister* were consistently depleted in individuals with depression, regardless of antidepressant treatment. *Faecalibacterium* and other *Coprococcus* species were consistently associated with better quality-of-life indicators.

Research linking neurotransmitters, brain activity, and the microbiome in humans is sparse. Animal subjects have been used for the most part. Since animals are not as adept as humans in communication, the classic "How does this make you feel?" approach normally used to monitor depression is lacking. But because we know the gut-brain axis exists, it is only a matter of time before we know if there are ways to improve mood disorders and mental illness with changes in gut microbes.

For more information, refer to "Anxiety, Depression, and the Microbiome: A Role for Gut Peptides" by Lach, Schellekens, Dinan, and Cryan, 2018:

> . . . we summarize the potential interactions of the microbiota with gut hormones and endocrine peptides, including neuropeptide Y, peptide YY, pancreatic polypeptide, cholecystokinin, glucagon-like peptide, corticotropin-releasing factor, oxytocin, and ghrelin in microbiome-to-brain signaling. Together, gut peptides are important regulators of microbiota-gut-brain signaling in health and stress-related psychiatric illnesses.

CHAPTER 13

CANCER CONCERNS

"Cancer is tough. Even saying it, it's a tough word to say."
—Luis Fonsi, Puerto Rican singer, songwriter, and actor

Cancer is the second leading cause of death in the United States. According to the World Health Organization, ninety-one of 172 countries polled ranked cancer as either the first or second most prevalent cause of death by age seventy.

As mentioned in the previous chapter, cancer is often a result of chronic inflammation and irritation (Balkwill & Mantovani, 2002; Coussens & Werb, 2001). Studies estimate that about 15 percent of cancers worldwide are associated with microbial infection (Kuper, Adami, & Trichopoulos, 2000). The bacterium *H. pylori*, which causes stomach cancer, is one example. We also know that cancer can be a result of viral infections like the human papilloma virus, which can lead to cervical cancer.

There is another piece to the cancer/inflammatory puzzle. Anti-inflammatory drugs (NSAIDS) have been shown to suppress tumors in people with familial adenomatous polyposis (FAP), an inherited disorder characterized by cancer of the colon and rectum.

It is also thought that chronic inflammation, irritation, and infection leads to cell death and the body must have a way to repair itself. In the early stages of tumors, the body treats them much like wounds that need healing. Our immune system may be attempting this repair when things go wrong—like genetic mutations. The lesion itself has reprogrammed the genetic pathway. The healing process then speeds out of control like a runaway train. Too many cells are produced, which causes tumors to develop. And it is in later stage that the tumors themselves appear to be driving the train, causing more inflammation (Coussens, et al., 1999).

For many years, researchers have suspected that microbiota played a part in the signaling process that determined if inflammation led to cancer. There are many microbial "pattern recognition receptors" for detecting viruses and bacteria (Meylan, Tschopp, & Karin, 2006). In other words, certain microbes recognize bacteria and viruses in their environment.

Pushalkar, et al. (2018) found that a cancerous pancreas harbors a distinctly abundant microbiome compared with the normal pancreas in both mice and humans, and certain bacteria are increased in the cancerous pancreas compared with gut. In fact, *Proteobacteria* are less than 10 percent of the gut bacteria of pancreatic ductal adenocarcinoma patients but they increased to 50 percent in the cancerous pancreas. The researchers also found that in mice, the use

> **PD-1** is protein found on T cells (a type of immune cell) that modulates the body's immune responses. When PD-1 is bound to another protein called PD-L1, it helps keep T cells from killing other cells, including cancer cells. Some anticancer drugs, called immune checkpoint inhibitors (ICIs), are used to block PD-1.

of antibiotics halted disease progression and the reintroduction of the bacteria accelerated tumor growth.

Researchers have also found that the presence of the bacteria *Akkermansia muciniphilia* increases the response to immunotherapy, a biologic treatment that boosts the body's natural defenses to fight cancer, in some cancer patients (Routy, et al., 2017). Other researchers (Matson, et al., 2018; Gopalakrishnan, et al., 2017) found that patients who responded favorably to the immunotherapeutic PD-1 drug (PD stands for programmed cell death) also had a greater abundance of "good" bacteria.

Some researchers have found increased risk for esophageal, gastric, and pancreatic cancers with previous penicillin treatment (Boursi, Mamtani, Haynes, and Yang, 2015). Lung cancer risk also increased with the use of penicillin. Incidentally, the researchers found no association between use of anti-virals and anti-fungals and cancer risk.

All of this leads us to the thread of insight that our microbiome plays a role in inflammation and disease and that reducing inflammation may be the first step in preventing disease. And protecting our microbiome might be the first step in preventing inflammation.

CHAPTER 14

WHAT TO AVOID

"A smart man makes a mistake, learns from it, and never makes that mistake again. But a wise man finds a smart man and learns from him how to avoid the mistake altogether."
—Roy H. Williams

Healthy choices depend heavily on the individual. Because everyone is different, there are few foods that make the universal food choice list. However, there are several things that seem to consistently cause stomach distress and others that are just unhealthy. Eventually, we will know how these things affect our microbiome and why some people tolerate them better than others.

Corn is on my do-not-try list. If you read the chapter on gas, you know that corn in any form doesn't digest, is over genetically modified, and doesn't provide much in the way of nutritional value. Microwave popcorn has carcinogens and popped corn in general is irritating to the lining of the digestive tract.

Raw salads and **raw vegetables** are another food that people over forty with slower digestion should probably avoid. It takes a lot of digestive energy to process lettuce and raw spinach, and you are more likely to be sickened by pathogenic bacteria (food poisoning). Because raw vegetables sit in the gut for so long, they collect more microbiota and are likely to cause an overgrowth of bacteria (SIBO). Eating raw is not for everyone. Especially

SYMPTOMS OF FOOD POISONING:
- Nausea
- Vomiting
- Diarrhea—watery or bloody
- Cramps
- Fever

avoid raw foods with a lot of insoluble fiber like asparagus, celery, zucchini, broccoli, leafy greens, and root vegetables. Cooking is key. Try steaming or grilling.

Smoking **cigarettes** and **cigars** contribute to heartburn and indigestion. One problem is that tobacco inhibits the production of saliva, impeding the breakdown of food. Smokers are also more likely to have gum disease because of this.

People who suffer with acid reflux, heartburn, or GERD should avoid chocolate, caffeine, and alcohol. **Chocolate** causes intestinal cells to release serotonin which relaxes the esophageal sphincter causing gastric contents to rise. Chocolate also contains caffeine and theobromine, which increases symptoms. Some people cannot tolerate the acid in **coffee** or tea and the added caffeine can increase gut motility to the point that important nutrients are not absorbed. Even small amounts of **alcohol** can irritate your stomach by making it produce too much acid, causing gastritis.

Greasy foods and fried foods (which includes many fast foods) also lead to reflux because they prevent the lower esophageal sphincter from closing. Heavier foods in general take longer to digest causing the stomach to empty more slowly which can also cause heartburn.

The **peppermint** sword cuts both ways. For some, peppermint tea is a soothing solution for indigestion or gas. For others, peppermint causes heartburn and GERD. This is because peppermint lowers esophageal pressure allowing reflux indigestion.

Tomatoes, tomato sauces, ketchup, marinara sauce, and tomato-based soups all have considerable amounts of acid and can easily aggravate GERD. People with diverticulitis are known to be sensitive to the seeds. However, tomatoes also contain lycopene (an antioxidant), so if you can tolerate tomatoes in any form—including raw—bon appétit.

Spicy foods are the bane of many. They often contain a compound called capsaicin. Capsaicin is both good and bad. It is an anti-inflammatory, which means that is good for arthritis; however, it can cause heartburn, indigestion, and even diarrhea. Sometimes it depends on the amount of capsaicin. Let's face it, not all hot sauces are created equal. But if your eyes start to water or your skin burns when you open the bottle, save your tissues the trouble. The honeymoon and the divorce may be painful.

Bacteria known to cause food poisoning:		
Name	*Onset*	*High-risk foods and practices*
Campylobacter	2–5 days	Meat and poultry, unpasteurized milk, and contaminated water.
Clostridium botulinum	12–72 hrs	Improperly canned foods, salted or smoked fish, potatoes cooked in aluminum foil, and foods kept at warm temperatures for too long.
Clostridium perfringens	8–16 hrs	Meats, stews, and gravies not kept hot enough or chilled too slowly.
Escherichia coli (E. coli) O157:H7	1–8 days	Feces-contaminated beef that is undercooked. Other sources include unpasteurized milk, apple cider, alfalfa sprouts, and water.
Giardia lamblia	1–2 weeks	Raw produce, infected food handlers, or contaminated water.
Hepatitis A	2–7 weeks	Raw produce, shellfish, or infected food handlers.

Listeria	9–48 hrs	Raw produce, processed meats, unpasteurized milk and cheeses, contaminated soil and water.
Noroviruses	12–48 hrs	Raw produce, shellfish from contaminated water or infected food handler.
Rotavirus	1–3 days	Raw produce and infected food handlers.
Salmonella	1–3 days	Meats, poultry, milk, or egg yolks. Survives inadequate cooking; can live on utensils and hands.
Shigella	24–48 hrs	Seafood, raw produce, and infected food handlers.
Staphylococcus aureus	1–6 hrs	Lives on skin: hand contact, coughing and sneezing. Meats and prepared salads, cream sauces, and cream-filled pastries.
Vibrio vulnificus	1–7 days	Raw and undercooked oysters, mussels, clams, and whole scallops.

CHAPTER 15

MONEY IN THE BANK

"Your diet is a bank account. Good food choices are good investments."
—Bethenny Frankel

There are several foods that deserve to make the tongue to tush trip. Some of them are as common as cats, others more exotic. I would be remiss if I didn't mention some favorites.

SWEET POTATO

Most colorful roots and tubers (beets, carrots, sweet potatoes, turmeric, and yams) are our friends—and I love sweet potatoes. But don't confuse sweet potatoes with their paler sibling, the yam. The sweet potato is an awesomely versatile vegetable that can be used in many different types of dishes: from starters, to entrees, to desserts.

> **Yam vs. Sweet Potato** Yams have darker and sometimes rougher skin. Yams are drier and require more oil, cream, or butter when cooked, and have more starch than sweet potatoes. Sweet potatoes are naturally sweeter and do not require as many ingredients for them to be tasty and have fewer calories.

I mix flavors and make a nice casserole using sweet potatoes, apples, and nuts.

Sweet potatoes are a high source of fiber and low in gas production. They are also rich in vitamin A, vitamin B6, and potassium.

SWEET POTATO WEDGES
Scrub sweet potatoes. Cut into wedges.
Place on shallow pan. Sprinkle with season salt, pepper, and chili powder. Drizzle with olive oil.
Cook at 400°F for 20–25 minutes.

SPINACH

Spinach is a very good source of many different vitamins and minerals. You know it, I know it, your mom knows it, Popeye knows it. But raw spinach happens to be very low in fiber, which, in turn, means that your body will accumulate more gas when you consume it.

I love a good spinach salad, but in moderation. Raw spinach is high in vitamin A, but eating cooked spinach increases the absorption of vitamins A and E, protein, fiber, zinc, thiamin, calcium, and iron. Important carotenoids, such as beta-carotene, lutein, and zeaxanthin, also become more absorbable.

Spinach can be sautéed in olive oil with garlic and lightly salted for a quick side dish. Cook for about a minute after it starts to simmer. Some people sprinkle it with parmesan cheese and others recommend the squeeze of a lemon.

SIMPLE SPINACH CASSEROLE

2 16-oz packages of fresh baby spinach, washed

5 Tbsp butter

3 Tbsp olive oil

2–3 cloves garlic, minced

¾ tsp salt

1 Tbsp Italian seasoning

1 cup grated Parmesan cheese

Preheat oven to 400°. In a stockpot, bring 5 cups water or broth to a boil. Add washed spinach; cover and cook for 1 minute or until wilted. Drain. In a small skillet, heat butter and oil over medium-low heat. Add garlic, Italian seasoning, and salt; cook and stir until garlic is tender, 1–2 minutes. Spread spinach in a greased 1-½-qt. baking dish. Drizzle with butter mixture; sprinkle with cheese. Bake, uncovered, until cheese is lightly browned, for 10–15 minutes.

BEET

The leaves of the beet plant have been eaten for decades, but not until the 1800s were beets considered a delicacy when the roots were made popular by French chefs. Not only do they have a satisfying crisp texture, but they can color your pee an exciting shade of red.

Beets can be eaten raw, steamed, boiled, baked, sautéed, pickled, etc.—the list is longer than your intestine. In Australia, pickled beets are served on hamburgers. Beets are good for digestion and low in gas production. Beets are a good source of folate, and cooked beets are high

COOKING FOOD CAN:

- Increase bioavailability of lycopene in tomatoes.
- Increase bioavailability of beta carotene in sweet potatoes, tomatoes, carrots, and spinach.
- Increase absorption of iron and other minerals by decreasing oxalates.

in vitamin C and a good source of riboflavin. Research suggests that nitrates from vegetables like beets lowers blood pressure and increases athletic performance.

Since beets' phytonutrients are diminished by heat, I recommend steaming beets for fifteen minutes or until they are cooked *al dente*. They can also be sautéed or roasted in garlic and olive oil with sweet potatoes, carrots, and fennel for a healthy delicious main course. Toss in a bit of thyme for balance.

ROASTED BEET SALAD

4 medium red beets	½ tsp paprika
Juice of half a lemon	2 Tbsp olive oil
Juice of half an orange	¼ tsp salt
1. Tbsp balsamic vinegar	Pinch of fresh-ground pepper
1 clove garlic, minced	3 Tbsp chopped cilantro
½ tsp ground cumin	

Wash beets and place on foil-lined baking sheet. Bake at 350°F for an hour or until fork tender. Cool, peel, and cut into bite-sized pieces. For vinaigrette, puree one cooked beet with the lemon and orange juice, balsamic vinegar, garlic, cumin, paprika, olive oil, salt, and pepper. (Can be done the day before.) Before serving, toss the beets with vinaigrette. Garnish with fresh cilantro.

CARROT

Bugs Bunny had a lot more going on than preventing eye ailments when he chomped on carrots. Not only do these root vegetables add a dash of color to whatever dish you're preparing, but they also have numerous health benefits. I love using carrots in baked cakes and muffins. It's a bit different than their conventional use and they add a unique and sweet flavor to any dish. Carrots are a good source of fiber and low in gas production. According to *Scientific American*, "Fact or Fiction: Raw Veggies are Healthier than Cooked Ones," there is research that cooked carrots have higher levels of beta-carotene than the raw ones, which our body converts into vitamin A. Try them roasted and lightly covered in a couple of tablespoons of olive oil sprinkled with garlic, oregano, basil, parsley, thyme, salt, and pepper. Cook at 375° until fork tender.

CARROT TOSS

Mix olive oil, garlic, Parmesan, breadcrumbs, salt, and pepper. Toss all ingredients together with cut carrots. Spread out and bake at 400° for 20–25 minutes or until tender. Turn with a spatula halfway through.

ARTICHOKE

Look for artichokes with tightly packed thick leaves and dark green color. While you probably think of drizzling hollandaise sauce over this tasty vegetable, there are other preparations that are drastically healthier. After peeling the pulpy scales of the artichoke, the tender "heart" of the plant may be added to sauces, pasta dishes, pizzas, and green salads to add a bit of a nutty flavor. Although this vegetable is very high in fiber, high in vitamin C, and a good source of folate, it's a notorious gas producer—not Tinder first-date fare (unless you really should've swiped left). Artichokes boiled for ten to twelve minutes can be halved, then grilled with garlic, parsley, and olive oil for a tasty and nutritious side dish.

CABBAGE

Cabbage has been used as an herbal medicine—as well as in food—for years. The workers who built the Great Wall of China were actually fed cabbage to keep them strong and healthy during the laborious process. Cabbage is healthy for many reasons. It is full of vitamin K and anthocyanins that help with mental function and prevent nerve damage, improving your defense against Alzheimer's disease and dementia.

Because it is low in calories and high in fiber, cabbage is a good weight loss

> ## HOMEMADE SAUERKRAUT
> Combine shredded cabbage with some salt and pack it into a jar—or crock if you want to make a lot. Mason jars work fine for small batches. The cabbage releases liquid, creating its own brining solution. Submerged in this liquid for a period of several days or weeks, the cabbage slowly ferments into the crunchy, sour condiment we know and love as sauerkraut.

food and helps to cleanse the body when it's too acidic. Cabbage can be good for healing ulcers and heartburn. Cabbage also acts as a mild laxative. Cabbage is used to flush out and cleanse the system when eaten, and the leaves can be applied externally to reduce swelling. Naturopaths claim it can be helpful for strain, sprains, bursitis, bruises, and breast engorgement.

Both French and English cuisine associate various cabbage dishes with home and hearth. In French, the phrase, "mon petit chou," which means "my little cabbage," is a term of endearment for children.

Sauerkraut is a very healthy form of cabbage. It contains far more *lactobacillus* than yogurt. You can ferment it at home in a jar.

FENNEL

You may be acquainted with licorice-flavored fennel seeds. However, the most nutritious part of fennel is the bulb. A single bulb has plenty of iron, fiber, and potassium, and 20 percent of your daily vitamin C.

Native to the Mediterranean region, most fennel in American markets is grown in California. Florence fennel resembles celery. Fennel can be grilled, roasted, or sautéed. And remember, fennel is also excellent for reducing gas.

FENNEL & FISH ENTRÉE

1 tsp crushed fennel seeds

¼ cup room temp. butter

2 Tbsp minced shallots

2 Tbsp chopped fennel fronds

1 fennel bulb

7 ounces salmon fillets

2 Tbsp anise-flavored liqueur

In large nonstick skillet, stir fennel seeds over medium heat until fragrant, about 1½ min. Move to small bowl. Add butter, shallots, 1 tablespoon fennel fronds, and season with salt and pepper. Melt 1 tablespoon of the butter mixture in the large nonstick skillet over medium heat. Add sliced fennel bulb and ¼ cup water. Cover and cook for about 8–10 minutes until crisp-tender. Uncover and sauté until fennel begins to brown. Transfer fennel to plate. Salt and pepper salmon, melt 1 tablespoon butter mixture in skillet over medium heat. Add salmon, cover and cook for 5 minutes. Turn salmon over, add ¼ cup water to skillet. Cover and continue cooking (about 5 minutes) until salmon is opaque in center. Move salmon to side of skillet, return fennel to skillet. Add 2 teaspoon butter, liqueur, and remaining fronds. Stir & heat through.

YOGURT

Since yogurt is fermented, it's good for your gut. Check labels for the National Yogurt Associations (NYA) Live and Active Cultures seal to ensure you are getting the bacteria you paid for. Always look for low-fat yogurts without added sugars. Yogurt is a good source of calcium, protein, vitamin B12, phosphorus, riboflavin B2, and potassium. Greek yogurts usually have twice or more the amount of protein than regular yogurts.

FERMENTED LEMONS

Moroccan Preserved Lemons are a treat. Their citrus and salty notes ferment into unique complex flavor that's delicious with fish, chicken, and grilled or roasted vegetables. The rind softens and becomes quite delectable. Fermented lemons may be good for those with bacterial overgrowth and could be a good cleanse. No one will conduct a million-dollar clinical trial to investigate the benefits of fermented lemons. You will just have to trust my expertise as a gastroenterologist and fermented lemon lover.

FERMENTED LEMONS

Start with 5 organic lemons and cut the bumps off each end. Cut lengthwise into quarters leaving about ¼ of the ends attached. Sprinkle a teaspoon of salt into a pint jar. Sprinkle another teaspoon inside the quartered lemon.

End down, stuff the lemon into the jar and squish it. Sprinkle on another teaspoon of salt. Repeat until the jar is full and stuff as much as possible. You can squeeze more juice into the jar until it is half full of lemon juice.

(Continue on next page)

Screw on the lid, let sit at room temperature for three days, give it a shake, and turn it upside-down and then right-side up a few times a day. After three days, place the jar in the refrigerator and let it sit for three weeks before using. Store in refrigerator.

Discard the pulp—it's the peel that is used. Wash the peel thoroughly to remove excess salt.

JICAMA

This yellow tuber is also known as Mexican turnip. Its inside is a creamy white texture that resembles raw potato or pear. The flavor is sweet and starchy, and it is usually eaten raw, sometimes with salt, paprika, and lemon or lime. It can be cut into slices and dipped in salsa. It is also cooked in soups and stir-fried dishes.

KEFIR

People used to drink soured milk—milk with natural bacteria left unrefrigerated to ferment. Now we prefer a fermented milk drink with a sour taste, made with a culture of yeasts and bacteria. Kefir has beneficial yeast as well as probiotic bacteria. The name Kefir comes from the Turkish word *keyif*, which means "good feeling." Kefir is known to reduce levels of the bacteria *H. pylori* in the stomach. Kefir has also been shown to improve *C. diff* infections (Spinler et al., 2016).

You can make it at home by adding active kefir grains (kefir starter) into four cups of fresh milk. Cover with a coffee filter secured by a rubber band or jar ring. Place in a warm spot, 68°–85°F, to culture.

MANUKA HONEY

Native to New Zealand and Australia, manuka honey is produced by bees that pollinate the flower *Leptospermum scoparium* or the manuka bush. Manuka honey is rich in the compound Methylglyoxal that is believed to be a powerful antiviral, anti-inflammatory, and antibacterial component. In 2007, it was approved by the US FDA for wound treatment. It has also been proven to treat gingivitis, sore throats, gastric ulcers, IBS, acne, and even symptoms of cystic fibrosis. Manuka honey has been used successfully to reduce *C. diff* bacteria (Hammond & Donkor, 2013).

NATTO

This is a traditional Japanese food made from soybeans fermented with *Bacillus subtilis*. It is a tad sticky with a unique taste, texture, and smell. It takes a little getting used to. It can be eaten with rice, soy sauce or mentsuyu sauce (sake, mirin, light soy sauce, dried seaweed, and dried bonito flakes), Japanese mustard, and green onions.

NUTS

Nuts are high in nutritional value. One serving of mixed nuts has 12 percent of the Recommended Daily Intake of vitamin E, 16 percent of the RDI of magnesium, 13 percent of the RDI of phosphorus, 23 percent of the RDI of copper, 23 percent of the RDI of manganese and 56 percent of the RDI of selenium. Select raw or dry roasted nuts whenever possible. Roasting nuts at too-high temperatures or in unstable oils may alter and damage the polyunsaturated (good fats) and contribute to the formation of the toxin acrylamide. Remember to chew, chew, and chew. Keep in mind that nuts may not be a good fit for those with diverticulosis. Research is always underway and influencing what we believe.

CHEESE

Not all cheese is created equal. While some avoid cheese because of the high fat content, cheese is healthy. It is high in protein, calcium, and several other nutrients.

Fermented cheese is far healthier than processed cheese. Look for mozzarella made from Italian buffalo or cow's milk. Mozzarella contains *Lactobacillus casei* and *Lactobacillus fermentum*.

Cheddar is a widely popular semi-hard cheese that originated in England. Cheddar is rich in vitamin K2.

Goat cheeses have more medium-chain fatty acids than those made from cow's milk.

Blue cheese can be made from cow, goat, or sheep's milk that has been cured with *Penicillium* (mold) cultures.

Feta was originally made in Greece. It is a soft, salty, white cheese usually made from sheep or goat's milk. Sheep's milk feta is tangy and sharp, while goat feta is mild. Feta can be high in sodium, but it is typically lower in calories than other cheeses.

KIMCHI

A staple in Korean cuisine, kimchi is made from salted and fermented vegetables, most commonly napa cabbage and Korean radishes, with a variety of seasonings, including gochugaru, scallions, garlic, ginger, and jeotgal. Koreans each consume about forty pounds of kimchi per year. It is thought to be high in the bacteria *Lactobacillus, Leuconostoc,* and *Weissella.* Because we all have different bacterial needs, kimchi may not suit everyone. Start slow and try a smaller amount to see if it is compatible with your unique microbiome.

CHAPTER **16**

FECAL FEAT

"In the early days of oral antibiotics, we were plagued by frequent diarrhea in our patients due presumably to killing off intestinal bacteria. I was Chief of Surgery at the VA and simplistically considered merely reintroducing normal organisms to counter such absence. Those were days when if one had an idea, we simply tried. It seemed to work, and I wrote it up. It made a small splash."

—Ben Eiseman, M.D.

Stool transplant is the process of taking stool (feces) from a healthy individual and implanting it into the colon of a diseased individual via colonoscopy, enema, nasogastric or nasojejunal tubes, capsules, or endoscopy.

Remember when you were a kid, and you were completely bored? Then a friend came over and everything that was old was new again. Your toys took on a whole different personality. Watching the same old cartoons had a fresh appeal. Maybe you even got into a bit of mischief? Think of a stool transplant, a.k.a. fecal microbiota transplant (FMT), as a stimulating play date.

This process introduces new bacteria, which reorganizes and reshapes our gut's bacterial populations. The new bacteria may reduce pathogenic (bad) bacteria and stimulate our immune systems. It may change the ratios of microbes that process food, store fat, or make energy. It may encourage important metabolic pathways that have waned.

Using feces as medicine is nothing new. As early as the fourth century, Chinese scholar Ge Hong (283–343 AD) penned a recipe for *yellow soup*, a broth made with dried or fermented stool from a healthy person. The broth was swallowed by mouth and resulted in healing. Don't mistake this primordial porridge for the delicious yellow saffron vegetable soups popular today—look for a nice, fresh garnish—although both are said to have a healing effect.

In the sixteenth century, Chinese physician, scientist, pharmacologist, herbalist, and acupuncturist, Li Shizhen (1518–1593) used a fermented fecal solution to treat fever, diarrhea, vomiting, and constipation.

A century later, veterinarians used fecal transplants to cure diarrhea in horses.

The first known fecal microbiota transplant in western medicine was in 1958 by Ben Eiseman (1917–2012) and colleagues. A team of surgeons from Colorado treated four critically ill people with what was called fulminant pseudomembranous colitis using fecal enemas, which resulted in rapid recovery. We now know *C. difficile* to be the cause of fulminant pseudomembranous colitis.

A significant advancement in fecal transplantation has been the use of frozen fecal matter. In 1998, researchers (Gustafsson, et al., 1999) in Sweden used frozen fecal matter to treat *C. diff.* The winter temperature in Stockholm gets as low as 5° F, so frozen feces was probably a natural fit. Since then, over a dozen researchers worldwide have used frozen feces in the treatment of *C. diff.* Studies have found viability in frozen feces for up to one year in storage. I strongly recommend that you consult with a gastroenterologist who *specializes in FMT* before considering any fecal treatment/therapy.

Upper gastrointestinal routes of FMT include nasal tubes (up your nose with a rubber hose) that lead to the stomach or the small intestine and oral capsules that are either fresh, frozen, or freeze-dried. These methods can be faster and less expensive.

> A **nasojejunal tube** is a soft, slim tube that is put in through the nose, through the stomach, and ends in the jejunum—a part of the small intestine.

Common lower gastrointestinal methods include colonoscopy and enemas. There are benefits and pitfalls for each type of procedure. Physicians will choose the one that best fits a combination of availability, their patients' needs, and/or their own expertise.

The major advantage that colonoscopy offers over other modalities is the ability to see the entire colon and shop for the best fit for a transplant. There is also the possibility of better retention of the transplanted stool. A colonoscopy can deliver larger amounts of stool per procedure and is associated with consistently higher success rates.

Enemas are easier. FMT via enema can be done in the hospital or the doctor's office. However, access to parts of the colon that are the most receptive to new bacteria may not be available and patients with poor sphincter tone may not be able to hold the enema long enough for successful **refloralization**.

> **Refloralization** is my own term for bringing back the flora (more diverse bacteria, fungi) into the colon. The process can involve placing feces directly into the cecum or simply providing nutrients needed to grow missing microbes in the colon. The latter process would attempt to bring the balance back in the microbiome without the need for stool donors.

In 2013, a review and meta-analysis in the *American Journal of Gastroenterology* demonstrated that FMT done by a gastroenterologist testing their donors resolved nearly 90 percent of recurrent *C. Diff* infection. While there have been some side effects like fever, flatulence, bloating, nausea, vomiting, abdominal pain, and constipation reported immediately after FMT, the other more serious health considerations are discussed in the next chapter.

As of the date of this writing, the Food and Drug Administration has only approved FMT for the treatment of recurrent *C. diff* and nothing else. But innovative entrepreneurs have not let this stop them. There are capsules of poop that can be bought and swallowed. There are online directions and YouTube videos for do-it-yourself enemas. Poop can be purchased, sold, and traded like any commodity. There are even lists of those claiming to be superior donors. But unless you have lost all hope in the health-care system, my advice is to leave FMT (and tattoos) to the experts. There are many reasons why amateurs and DIYers could go wrong in fecal transfers. Even play dates need adult supervision.

The oral capsules that claim to contain fecal microbiota have not shown to be as effective in treating *C. diff* as a personalized approach Many intestinal bacteria don't survive for long outside the body. The intestine's important anerobic bacteria is especially sensitive, so the likelihood of receiving the specific healthy bacteria ratio you might need is low.

However, in a 2017 issue of JAMA (*Journal of American Medical Association*) there is a report of oral capsules used successfully for FMT. Kao, et al., (2017) conducted medically supervised trials and found oral capsular FMT equal to that of direct implantation to the cecum via colonoscopy. The fecal microbes in the study were obtained from frozen donor poop, processed to only contain bacteria and delivered to the subject in a relatively short period of time. However, later follow-up observations found no long-term benefits for subjects.

Until we know more about the number of FMTs that might be required for a particular disease, or we have more research on what types of patients are better suited for the different delivery methods, my advice is to proceed with caution and read the next chapter.

Chapter 17

TRANSPLANTATION COMPLICATION

"Truth is much too complicated to allow anything but approximations."
—John Von Neumann, mathematician

What could possibly go wrong? Transplanting feces and all of the bacteria, viruses, and fungi that it contains is not without risks. We know from blood transfusions that it is possible to transfer hepatitis C and HIV. It is possible that FMT recipients could receive microbes that could result in a disease rather than cure a disease?

There are a few isolated incidences where *C. diff* patients complained of weight gain after receiving FMT from obese biological donors. There might be a genetic precursor for obesity that was activated by the new microbiota. These cases have not been common, nor have they been investigated for other causes of weight gain, but theoretically, if we can cure with FMT, we can also cripple. Unfortunately, as of the date of this writing, there have been three deaths attributed to FMT.

There have also been cases in which recipients report arthritic symptoms after FMT. Some have also suggested that FMT administered via a nasogastric tube could be associated with increased risks of gastrointestinal bleed, peritonitis, and enteritis (Moayyedi, 2014).

Despite the robust research that links microbiome changes to different diseases, there are very few studies explaining the bio-chemical mechanisms responsible for the success

Peritonitis is inflammation of the peritoneum (a membrane lining the abdomen and covering the abdominal organs) usually caused by bacterial infection either via the blood or by a rupture.

Enteritis is an inflammation of the intestine, especially the small intestine, often accompanied by diarrhea.

of microbiome intervention. Although the rate of adverse post-FMT events appears to be low, no extensive research has formally sought out adverse diseases after FMT. Have we missed something? Do we need more research on the metabolic pathways that different microbiomes either alter or affect before FMT is considered a treatment option? Always discuss the risks versus benefits with your doctor before any health decision. Be a skeptic. Ask questions. All of us must be sentries of our own wellness.

Could I give a fecal recipient lymphoma? Could I cause a disease worse than the one I hoped to cure? There is also reason to believe that donor bacteria could be a key player. Read the next chapter: Who's Your Donor?

CHAPTER 18

WHO'S YOUR DONOR?

"You have not lived today until you have done something for someone who can never repay you."
—**John Bunyan,** *The Pilgrim's Progress*

Traditionally, fecal donors have been healthy biological relatives. Siblings, cousins, or parents were called to *doody*. It made sense. Relatives as donors shared similar genes, environments, and diets, so they probably shared a similar microbiome. And, they owed us. They were family. A shared environment also reduced the risk of transferring infectious agents to the recipient (Garborg, et al., 2010). Spousal donors put taking sh!t from your spouse to another level. I always advise to be nice to your spouse because you never know when you will need their sh!t, literally.

However, "Overall, current evidence indicates that the success of FMT does not depend on the donor-patient relationship; larger studies should be designed to explore this area in greater detail," (Ramai, et al., 2018). Some research found that unrelated blood donors selected by recipients were more likely to test positive for infectious disease markers than related donors (Starkey, et al., 1989), so asking friends for a donation is not without problems.

But it does avoid unpleasant phone conversations with your family. For example: You place a call to your healthiest relative, Auntie Marge, who has never been sick a day in her life and runs marathons for fun. She picks up on the second ring.

"Hello."

"Hey, Auntie Marge."

"Good to hear from you, dear. What's up? Anything new?"

Her cheery voice lifts your spirits.

"I'm so glad you asked. I was just wondering if you might be willing to give me some sh!t?" You give yourself a point for cleverness.

Silence.

You keep talking. "My doctor says that your poop might help get me out of the hospital."

More silence. Auntie Marge takes a deep breath and pulls the phone away.

"George, we're getting another one of those prank calls. . . ."

"No, Auntie Marge, it's me, your favorite niece—"

Click. Auntie Marge is not taking any crap. Nor is she giving any.

YOU ARE NOT ALONE

When 183 patients were asked about FMT donors, 28 percent of them found selecting their

> **BLOOD TESTS FOR DONORS:**
> - CBCWD
> - CMET
> - CMV IgG
> - CRE
> - EBV Ab Panel
> - Entamoeba histolytica
> - Hepatitis A, B, & C
> - HHV-6 IgG
> - HIV Antibody
> - HSV 1 & 2 IgG
> - HTLV-I/II Ab
> - IgE
> - Immunoglobulins Panel
> - JC Virus Ab
> - Lymphocyte Subset Panel
> - Strongyloides stercoralis
> - Syphilis
> - VRE

own donor too unappealing to consider FMT as a treatment (Zipursky, et al., 2012). Other researchers found when given a choice, all patients preferred stool from unknown donors (Hamilton, Weingarden, Sadowsky, & Khoruts, 2012). Obviously, we don't want someone we know giving us sh!t.

As of this writing, FMT outcomes from unknown donor stool are not statistically different than stool from biological relatives.

Fecal matter for FMT can be used fresh, or it can be frozen or freeze-dried and stored. To date, I know of no one who has attempted canning, but stool storage *is* an emerging field.

Recently, the use of stool banks has increased the use of unrelated donors. Terveer, et al. (2017) explains this in "How to: Establish and Run a Stool Bank." I'm sure, *Stool Banking for Dummies* is coming soon to a bookstore near you. This brings a whole new profession to the stage: What do you do for a living? Why, I'm a stool banker.

Stool banks are advantageous for those experiencing acute *C. difficile* colitis, since finding and screening suitable donors can take up to a week. Storing stool makes it immediately available and in the future, it may be available like blood products are today (Paramsothy, et al., 2015). The concept of stool banking does make one think that the future may not be in the bitcoin but in the sh!tcoin.

FREE TOASTERS?

We collect and store stool from donors in my medical office. It is a tricky business. As soon as donor stool is exposed to air, the anerobic bacteria are stressed and may even die. For fecal matter to retain its bacterial richness it must be sealed and immediately frozen. Stool that has been properly handled and stored may be viable for up to a year (Staley, et al., 2017).

Sometimes a person's own stool is used for FMT. These analogous donors will donate stool when their disease is in remission and then receive the transplant when they experience a flare-up.

HOW DO WE PROTECT OUR STOOL RECIPIENTS?

By thoroughly screening all our donors, whether we are talking about Auntie Marge or a medical student looking for extra credit. We test blood and stool looking for bacteria, viruses, fungi, and blood cell counts. We also test for Methicillin-resistant *Staphylococcus aureus* (MRSA) via nasal swab. More testing is on the way, especially after the COVID crisis. Any time a new illness rears its head, we add to the screening process.

These protocols protect recipients, and their families and friends. It can also be helpful to potential donors who may find out about an unknown health problem.

Ultimately, the perfect donor will be healthy with no known diseases. Their stool will have what we know to be healthy microbes in

STOOL TESTS/GI PANEL FOR DONORS:

- Adenovirus
- Astrovirus
- C. Diff
- Campylobacter
- Carbapenum (CRE)
- Covid-19
- Cryptosporidium
- Cyclospora cayetanensis
- E. Coli 0157
- Entamoeba histolytica
- Enteroaggregative E. coli
- Eneropathogenic E. coli
- Enterotoxigenic E. coli
- ESBL
- Giardia lamblia
- H. Pylori
- Norovirus GI/GII
- Plesiomonas
- Rotovirus A
- Salmonella
- Sapovirus
- Shig-like toxin E. coli
- Shigella/Entero E. coli
- Shigelloides
- Vibrio
- Vibrio cholera
- VRE

abundant numbers and rich in other lesser-known bacteria. I can only guess that in the not-so-distant future we may be able to transplant select bacteria as individual strains or as clusters known to improve a specific disease. Until then, we need to be vigilant about screening protocols and careful in our donor decisions.

HOW DO WE *DOO* IT?

Stool donations are non-invasive and take very little time. As we learn more about the different bacteria, we will be looking for specific donors who possess certain genera and species of microbiota. Eventually, it may be much like blood and tissue donations. Save a life, give someone sh!t.

CHAPTER 19

COLONOSCOPY CONSTERNATION

"If you get a colonoscopy, you should really insist they give you no drugs—
then you do get to see what it's like to swim through your own intestines."
—Mary Roach, humorist

Just when we thought our forties were challenging enough with teenagers, Spanx, and midlife crises, the United States Preventive Services Task Force (USPSTF) wants us to have our colons explored.

Colon cancer is the second leading cause of cancer death in the United States (Siegel, Naishadham, and Jemal, 2012). The risk of developing colon cancer increases at age forty-five. Europe, where colonoscopies aren't routine, is exploring the efficacy of routine colonoscopies. Randomized studies like the NordICC trial are under way in several countries.

Unfortunately, the results are a few years off. Until then, colonoscopies should be done every ten years or sooner if you are at increased risk. Anyone with polyps or first-degree biological relatives (parents, children, or siblings) who've had colon cancer should follow their doctor's advice for shorter interval testing.

Colonoscopies allow us to explore all of the colon and part of the small intestine via a small flexible camera. Fecal microbiota transplants are done using the same device and procedure.

But first we have to get all that waste out of the way. If I've done my job, you now know that human waste is really immunological gold. It's bacteria that keeps the human machine running like a recently updated iPhone.

I sense your hesitation. I've been selling microbiota like they were ocean front property in foreclosure and now I'm advocating eviction. Take a deep relaxing breath. Bacteria can replenish themselves at an incredible rate. Your amazing bacterial self will soon return.

We usually recommend that patients clear their bowels with a laxative preparation like bisacodyl, phospho soda, sodium picosulfate, or sodium phosphate and/or magnesium citrate) and large quantities of fluid the day before the scheduled colonoscopy. Yes, you might want to schedule the entire day at home. Up to 25 percent of all colonoscopies have inadequate bowel preparation (Froehlich, et al., 2005). So, unless you want the procedure repeated, follow your doctor's instructions. Some doctors will request a liquid diet of clear broth and lime or lemon Jell-O, others may ask you not eat after a certain time or a combination of both.

These are the same protocols we use for FMT. The bowels need to be clear before we introduce the new bacteria. It's a little like cleaning

COLONOSCOPY COMPLICATIONS:

- Reaction to sedative
- Bleeding from sites where a biopsy was taken, or a polyp or other abnormal tissue was removed
- Perforation to the colon or rectum wall
- Risk of complication during a colonoscopy is low, 0.35 percent.

before company comes but without the Swiffer. Because this evacuation does not kill bacteria *spores,* your own gut bacteria will rebound—unlike antibiotic therapy which also destroys spores.

In the USA, most colonoscopies are done with sedation. The use of anesthesia like midazolam, propofol, meperidine, and fentanyl administered by an anesthesiologist or a nurse anesthetist allows most patients to rest or sleep through the procedure. This is also the same protocol we use for FMT (via colonoscopy).

Many places around the world do not sedate or offer sedation for colonoscopies. Researchers found that out of eighty sedation-free colonoscopies: five required sedation to complete the colonoscopy, four experienced no pain, thirty-two had mild pain, twenty-seven experienced moderate pain, and sixteen had severe pain. When asked if they would choose the sedation-free colonoscopy again: fifty-eight were willing (Hoffman, Butler, & Shaver, 1998).

There is research that suggests sedation increases the risk of adverse events during a colonoscopy. One of the advantages of not being sedated is that the patient can alert the physician to any pain that might be related to pressure on the wall of the colon preventing perforation.

Patients are asked to lie on their left side during the procedure. Initially, I perform a rectal examination with a gloved hand, to examine the tone of the sphincter and to see if the preparation is sufficient. The endoscope is then passed through the anus to the rectum, the colon (sigmoid, descending, transverse, and ascending colon, the cecum), and ultimately to the end of the small intestine that connects to the large intestine.

The endoscope is a long tube divided into separate channels for instrumentation, air, suction, and light. The instrument has a small movable tip, less than 0.5 inches in diameter. The empty bowel is usually collapsed, so air is blown in to maximize visibility, which can also cause the false sensation of needing to poop.

Biopsies of suspicious areas are taken. Suspicious lesions may be cauterized, treated, or biopsied with an electric wire. We usually remove polyps that are one millimeter (0.04 of an inch) or less. It is rare that problems occur during a colonoscopy. Sometimes dye (indigo carmine) may be sprayed through the endoscope onto the bowel wall to see any abnormalities in the lining (chromoscopy).

Occasionally, (0.35 percent) a small perforation may occur, these will usually heal on their own. Rarely, a larger perforation will need to be surgically repaired.

The trip to the cecum, the junction of where the colon and small bowel join up, is usually less than ten minutes. Due to tight turns and roller-coaster redundancy, parts of the colon are loops that cause "bowing" of the endoscope, which causes the tip to retract. These loops can cause discomfort due to stretching. Usually, gently pulling the endoscope while twisting it will free it. Changes in body position and adding hand pressure can often straighten the endoscope, allowing it to move forward.

By the way, fecal transplants are implanted in the cecum, the hub of the microbiome. Donor stool is prepared as an aqueous solution and drawn into the endoscopic tube and deposited.

After your colonoscopy procedure, you will rest in the clinic or hospital while the anesthesia wears off. For most this usually takes an hour, but for some it can be longer. Someone must drive you home. Because of the possibility of lingering effects of anesthesia, it's advised that you don't make any important decisions for the rest of the day. This includes shopping for bathing suits.

A **polyp** is an abnormal growth that can appear on the lining of the colon (large intestine) that sticks out into the colon passageway.

Polyps can be raised or flat. It can take up to fifteen years for a polyp to turn cancerous.

CHAPTER 20

IS FMT FOR YOU?

"The consumption of 'fresh, warm camel feces' has also been recommended by Bedouins as a remedy for bacterial dysentery."
—Wikipedia

Even though feces have been used as cures for centuries, the US Food and Drug Administration (FDA) did not allow FMT until 2013 when they made a ruling that permitted doctors to provide FMT without filing the standard investigational New Drug Application (NDA) to treat recurrent *C. difficile* infection. As of this writing, fecal microbiota transplants are FDA allowed for no other disease. Of the five hundred thousand people in the US who are annually infected with *C. diff*, at least half will be re-infected. *C. diff*-related costs are over $5 billion a year, which does increase pressure for the FDA to formally approve FMT for the routine treatment of *C. diff*—before it recurs.

A two-year study sponsored by the American Gastroenterological Association's (AGA) fecal microbiota transplantation is currently underway. The research is planned to be the largest of its kind and may expand the scope of FMT and disease. The AGA registry plans to enroll seventy-five FMT sites and track four thousand patients for five to ten years after their FMT procedure.

However, FMT for other diseases may never be approved unless a standardized method of collection, storage, and delivery is established. It is likely that big pharma will be the first to produce FDA-approved microbiome products for particular diseases. Pharmaceutical companies are researching the possibilities, but hopefully it will remain with the doctor/patient relationship to decide what makes the best donor for a particular person.

Doctors are bound by these regulations. The FDA is our benevolent gatekeeper and prevents Dr. Frankenstein from setting up shop down the street and ruining property values for all of us. The FDA knows that anything that can cure can also kill. Since I have a clinical trial practice, I work with the FDA on a regular basis. I look to them for guidance and feel that their protocols allow us to face the future with courage rather than regret.

CHAPTER 21

THE FUTURE

"If we knew what it was we were doing, it would not be
called research, would it?"
—Albert Einstein

The more research I do, the more questions I have. When I was very
young, I might have asked, "Does this make my butt look big?"
Now, I find myself wondering if our hygienic culture has crippled our
microbiome. Are hand sanitizers and antibacterial products good or bad?
Researchers aren't sure. Do they prevent pathogens or promote bacterial
blitzkrieg?

We know that our Western high fat, highly processed food has
decreased our bacterial diversity. Will shipping these food products to
other cultures decrease their microbiome's bacterial richness? Are we
exporting metabolic syndrome?

Because we can eat food from all over the world, it exposes us to bacteria, fungi, and viruses we may never have been in contact with before.
Does our microbiome welcome these aliens or do they cause disease?

Most animal dung is richer and more diverse than human dung.
Are there microorganisms in other species that we might benefit from?

Elephants live long lives, seventy to eighty-six years. When you consider they survive outdoors, don't take medicine, and rarely have good internet—it's incredible. Is the secret in their microbiome?

Should we care for our microbiome? Are yogurt, fermented foods, and probiotics helpful in the long run? Do we take care of our microbiome, or does it take care of us? Until COVID, people were living longer than at any time in recorded history. Maybe our microbiome is already taking care of us.

I want you to think about the role of these millions of microorganisms. What if, instead of us *hosting* microorganisms, we are actually conduits for these life forms that may be older and more adaptable than we are? Bacteria may be the life force.

CHAPTER 22

DIRT TO DIRT

"Life is hard. Then you die. Then they throw dirt in your face. Then the worms eat you. Be grateful it happens in that order."

—David Gerrold, American science fiction writer

The process of aging increases our pathogenic bacteria. At death, that bad gut bacteria will eventually win, causing decomposition. But what happens to our microbiome then? It's a fair question. Humans have pondered the afterlife for eons. The Egyptians mummified everything: Baboons, cats, birds, and crocodiles—all hoping for another chance. Egyptians even preserved the intestines separately in canopic jars. But now that we are so worried about "contaminating" our water supplies and spreading disease, burial has become more sanitary—even sterile. We cremate.

Professor of Practice of Non-Fiction at Harvard University, Michael Pollan, recently wrote, "Some researchers believe that the alarming increase in autoimmune diseases in the West may owe to a disruption in the ancient relationship between our bodies and their 'old friends'–the microbial symbionts with whom we coevolved." The microbial symbionts he was writing about are the microorganisms in soil.

There are about forty million bacterial cells in one gram of soil. Up to fifty thousand species may exist in less than a teaspoon of soil. But agriculture has caused the mass destruction of our living soil environments and important species of microorganisms may have already gone extinct.

Actinobacteria are a diverse phylum of bacteria that exist in our water and in our soil. Many forms of plant life depend on them. *Actinobacteria* decompose organic matter and they fix nitrogen for plants to use. A Siberian strain is said to be one of the oldest living organisms on the planet. Types of *Actinobacteria* also live in our gut. Their ratios to other gut bacteria are low but they are imperative for homeostasis. Actinobacteria may be a co-evolutionary link between the soil and other life forms.

Perhaps part of our soil problem lies in burial practices that slow or prevent natural *refloralization.* If we are stripping the soil of microbes to produce food to feed the population, maybe the microbes that population produces should in turn feed the soil. Maybe a microbiome problem has a microbiome answer . . . .

Does our microbiota outlast us? Should our microbiome be allowed to re-enter the environment?

When we cremate, are we stealing from the ecosystem? Should our microbiome have a designated recycling number?

Natural burials or green burials allow bacteria to either die in peace or continue as part of a larger biome. Burial vaults are not allowed for green burials, but coffins made from materials that readily biodegrade may be used. In Israel, Jews are interred without a casket in a simple cloth shroud. Green burials also don't use embalming chemicals like formaldehyde (FA) which pollutes groundwater, poisoning fish. In 2004, The International Agency for Research on Cancer (IARC) classified FA as a human carcinogen. Embalmers must wear respirators because FA is toxic. Unfortunately, the impact of formaldehyde on our microbiome has yet to be explored in the context of human death.

Natural burials allow our bacterial flora that has come from the earth to return to the earth, to rekindle the cycle of life—or as the Egyptians believed—to be reborn.

IN CONCLUSION

While there is a vast chasm of unknown knowledge about the microbiome, and the role of bacteria on our health, I would like to review some conclusions based on what I have found so far.

Although every individual has a microbiome that is as unique as a fingerprint, we do understand that there may be a few consistent varieties or enterotypes. We also know that many healthy individuals have a different bacterial profile than their unhealthy, suffering counterparts. Research has shown that people with autism, heart disease, chronic constipation, inflammatory bowel disease, arthritis, and other illnesses have lower amounts of some bacteria and higher amounts of other bacteria, a condition that scientists have labeled dysbiosis.

We also know that diet, genetics, and environment play roles in our bacterial numbers—factors that contribute to our microbiome uniqueness. Antibiotics have also played a role in our microbial numbers. In the twentieth century, military-like assaults were made on microbes and infectious diseases. Unfortunately, overuse of antibiotics may have lowered our bacterial diversity and contributed to certain disease states.

Research has shown that fecal transplants are the answer to some infectious diseases like recurring *C. diff* infections and that ongoing studies will breach some of the barriers we are now facing.

Researchers are looking for ways to use this knowledge to explore the curative role of bacteria in other diseases hallmarked by dysbiosis.

Independent doctors have used FMT to improve several cases of colitis, constipation, Crohn's disease, Parkinson's, and autism, etc.

However, this type of idiopathic research does not have the strength of double-blind clinical trial research.

The human mind can be a confounding factor in healing. Asking subjects how they feel is not the same as longitudinal blood and fecal tests. How improvements are measured is subject to scientific rigor. Looking at improvement and decline in observable and measurable ways are critical. Data about side effects and adverse events after FMT are also an important part of FDA approval. This diligence protects us all.

Microbiome research is being done at an incredible pace and the technology to develop better capsules of poop that show high efficacy for *C. diff* is coming fast. More importantly doctors and scientists are realizing the importance of our microbiome in diseases. As we discover new microbes, cures are a possibility. What I write this year may change next year. The excitement over the possibilities is palpable in the medical care industry.

Because of this, I'm already planning and organizing my next book. *More Sh!t* is underway!

ACKNOWLEDGEMENTS

"No one who achieves success does so without acknowledging the help of others." —Alfred North Whitehead, philosopher

I could never have envisioned the possibility of FMT without the guidance and expertise of Dr. Sydney Finegold (1921–2018). Born to Russian immigrants, he was my professor, friend, and mentor. A UCLA graduate and WWII veteran, he then attended the University of Texas medical school in Galveston. He was one of the first scientists to posit a connection between anaerobes, infections, and autism.

It was Dr. Neil Stollman's search for a *C. diff* cure that planted the seeds of possibilities in my brain's backyard. His methodical and meticulous research as a gastroenterologist has been both grounding and inspiring. His words allowed me to understand the unfathomable and search for the unsearchable.

A special thank you goes to Thomas Borody, tireless researcher and patient sounding board. It was Dr. Borody's successful fecal transplants for Crohn's disease in Australia that bolstered my resolve to explore the possibilities outlined in this book.

A huge thank you to our determined copy editor, Kathleen Auth, who made this five-thousand-comma climb enjoyable and possible.

THE AUTHORS

"Dr. Hazan is an empathetic and intuitive physician, a brilliant
scientific researcher, and an inspiration and mentor to others. As a
fellow physician who collaborates on research with her, I can say she is
a valued colleague. In fact, I'm an authority on Sabine because she's also
my wife and mother of our children."
—Alon Steinberg, MD

Sabine Hazan was the first of four children born to two government
accountants in Morocco. In 1974, the family moved to Montreal,
Canada to provide better education and greater opportunities.

There, the Hazans raised their children with the ambition to match
their potential—all became doctors.

Throughout her life, Sabine's peers questioned her dream to become
a physician. But their challenges only fueled her ambitions. Even though
her primary language was French, she enrolled in Concordia University,
an English-speaking college.

Medical school admittance was difficult and more so for a woman.
Sabine was asked: What if you become pregnant? What would you do
if your child was sick, and you also had a sick patient needing care?
Whom would you choose? She wondered how many men were asked
such questions.

She graduated from Dalhousie Medical School in Halifax, Nova Scotia. Curious about the American healthcare system, she chose to do her residency in Internal Medicine at Jackson Memorial Hospital, a notoriously demanding and rigorous county hospital in Miami.

There, during the height of the HIV/AIDS crisis, she was under fire, learning to care for the most underserved patients who were desperately ill and dying. She fell further in love with medicine and with a fellow resident, whom she married in 1993.

During her early medical career, she was keenly interested in gastroenterology. "It's a man's specialty," she was told repeatedly. She would never be accepted. The naysayers again had the opposite effect and emboldened her resolve. In 1995, she became the first female Gastroenterology Fellow accepted at the University of Florida in Jacksonville. As a fellow, she discovered that she really enjoyed and excelled in clinical research, which led to awards from the university's Dean for Research as well as recognition from the American College of Physicians. At the time, her primary research was in esophageal diseases, part of her work with her formidable mentor, Dr. Sami Achem. Her husband, Dr. Alon Steinberg, completed his Cardiology Fellowship at the same time and the couple had their first daughter in 1996.

Following her fellowship, Dr. Hazan returned to Montreal and opened a practice across the border in upstate New York. Her enviable reputation grew quickly, and due to socialized medicine in Canada, long wait lists for procedures like colonoscopies brought in many Canadian patients in need of gastroenterology care.

Just as Apple and Tesla were visionaries of technology, Dr. Hazan pursued innovation in medicine. Some perceived her as a threat. A perfectionist in her scientific approach and focused in her quest for excellence, the multi-tasking Hazan was never one for bureaucracy and red tape. She was reported to the medical board, cited for poor record keeping, and required to take a course. The experience changed her. She became a warrior who vowed to extend her methodical approach in medical care to its documentation. In the ensuing years she emphasized extreme attention to detail, not just in her work product, but in her clinical research and records.

She now embraces oversight from the Food and Drug Administration (FDA) and Independent Review Board (IRB). Her clinical trials are known for their validation and verification.

After the couple's second daughter was born in 2004, Dr. Hazan rediscovered her passion for research and launched Ventura Clinical Trials. In 2005, she and her husband established respective patient practices in Ventura. Over the years, she attended several national GI conferences where she often met with her good friend and colleague, Dr. Neil Stollman, also a Gastroenterology Fellow in Miami during their residency years. Dr. Stollman had introduced her to the world of fecal microbiota transplant (FMT) and research being done by Dr. Thomas Borody since the late nineties.

Dr. Hazan started researching the use of FMT to treat patients with *C. diff*, which changed the trajectory of her career. It was Dr. Stollman's explorations that inspired her to consider the human digestive tract as the body's Garden of Eden. She later met Dr. Thomas Borody, the father of modern FMT. The meeting proved to be the beginning of a great collaborative relationship that continues to this day as they work together on advanced clinical research of the microbiome.

After hundreds of clinical trials and treating thousands of patients, Dr. Hazan still faced persistent questions about life, death, health, illness, the gut, and how they were connected. Various curiosities, innovative concepts, and ruminations kept her awake at night. Why did she crave McDonald's when she was pregnant the first time? Why does her first daughter still love it?

Alternatively, why does her youngest love vegetables, which Sabine craved often during her second pregnancy? Through research, she saw how dramatically the microbiome impacted human health, and she grew increasingly determined to understand.

Her curiosity led her to Dr. Sydney Finegold at UCLA. Dr. Finegold was certain of an association between bacteria, bowels, and behavior. He was especially sure of a connection between anaerobic bacteria and autism. If bacteria could contribute to autistic behavior, Dr. Hazan wondered if other tendencies, preferences, and characteristics could also be consequences of one's microbiome.

Could she study the bacteria in human feces and isolate it for treatment? Could she continue trailblazing through an emerging science? When preliminary research of the microbiome led to fecal material in capsules, with venture capitalists controlling the stocks of sh!t, one could say she went rogue. Strongly opposed to a "one pill fits all" solution, she felt called to pioneer her own microbiome research at the clinical level. She was determined to develop valid reproducible data and to leverage that data to emphasize the importance of individualized treatment for patients.

Resolute, she launched ProgenaBiome, a genetic sequencing research company dedicated to understanding the gut flora at the clinical level to advance FMT and other microbial-based therapies. As her professional network grew, she realized that doctors and researchers worldwide were asking the same questions. She traveled, addressed medical forums, and wrote articles in her quest for answers. Meanwhile, she worked persistently to help patients with celiac disease, Crohn's, ulcers, colitis, and other digestive ailments that she hypothesized were caused by dysbiosis in the gut.

Dr. Sabine Hazan's quest continues. She and Dr. Borody believe that answers to many medical mysteries and the power to heal may be within the trillions of microbes in the gut flora. Answers are close.

Science junkie **Sheli Ellsworth** grew up on a small farm in Texas and has seen both ends of the life cycle.

She graduated magna cum laude from Texas Woman's University and obtained her master's degree from West Texas A&M with concentrations in psychology and biology.

After three cases of food poisoning, a son who licked the floor to gross out his sister, and a poop-eating pug—she too had questions about bacteria, behavior, and why she continues ordering chicken enchiladas.

A humorist at heart, this is her seventh book. If you enjoy Sheli's writing, *Confessions of a Pet Au Pair*, an amusing guide to pet health, is available on Amazon.

Microbiome pioneer **Thomas Borody** was born in Krakow, Poland. His father, Jan Borody, fought in the defense of Warsaw during the Nazi invasion of 1939, and then his parents then survived the German occupation of Poland.

Jan, a pastor, worked as a double agent for the Polish underground while his photographer mother, Danuta, fed children trying to escape via sewage pipes from the ghetto.

His father found a way to take young Jewish girls out of ghettos and relocate them to the Krakow Carmelite nunnery where they could ultimately walk in groups over mountains to Switzerland and freedom. In Dec 1959, the family emigrated to Australia and settled in Sydney, where all three Borody children completed their medical training.

Edith became a family physician, Ian an obstetrician/ gynecologist, and Tom a gastroenterologist.

He completed his BS and MB BS degrees at the University of New South Wales then received his MD from Garvan Institute of Medical Research and University of Sydney School of Veterinary Science. He gained experience in parasitology, the treatment of TB and leprosy in the Solomon Islands, then spent three years in clinical research at the

Mayo Clinic, Rochester, MN. Later he earned a PhD at the University of Newcastle and his DSc at University of Technology Sydney.

Dr. Borody's clinical interests focus on the development of novel treatments including those of human gut microbiome using fecal microbiota transplantation (FMT) to treat *C. difficile* infection, colitis, irritable bowel syndrome as well as neurologic and autoimmune disorders. In 1984, Dr. Borody established the Centre for Digestive Diseases (CDD) in Sydney, Australia and has overseen its growth into an active clinical research institute with sixty-nine employees and twelve physicians treating around ten thousand patients per year. To date, Dr. Borody's clinic has completed some thirty-five thousand FMT treatments. He refined FMT by developing lyophilized (freeze-dried) FMT capsules and has published more than 310 research papers and has filed over 170 patents. His first FMT in 1988 was carried out on a patient with colitis who remained symptom free.

In 1985, he developed the first effective triple antibiotic therapy for *H. pylori*, which had a profound impact on curing hundreds of patients. The medication was sold in the US as Helidac.

He later licensed quadruple antibiotic therapy, now marketed as Pylera. He also developed the next generation, FDA-approved treatment for resistant *H. pylori*, Talicia.

Dr. Borody has also developed a Crohn's disease treatment now in pivotal trials, as well as colonoscopy bowel prep products Glycoprep, Glycoprep C, Moviprep, and a capsule prep licensed to Salix.

Future Borody therapies include asthma-reversing treatment and a product to treat coronary heart disease as chronic infection. He is currently focusing on the eradication of coronavirus using repurposed, combined anti-viral therapy.

REFERENCES

Agrawal, G., Borody, T.J., & Chamberlin, W. (2014). 'Global warming' to Mycobacterium avium subspecies paratuberculosis. *Future Microbiology*, 9(7), 829-832.

Ahmadmehrabi, S. & Tang, W. (2017). Gut microbiome and its role in cardiovascular diseases. *Current Opinion in Cardiology*, (6):761-766. doi: 10.1097/HCO.0000000000000445.

Ali, T., Lam, D., Bronze, M., & Humphrey, M. (2009). Osteoporosis in Inflammatory Bowel Disease. *American Journal of Medicine*, 122(7): 599–604. doi: 10.1016/j.amjmed.2009.01.022.

Allegretti, J., Kassam, Z., Mullish, B., Chiang, A., Carrellas, M., . . . Thompson, C. (2019). Effects of Fecal Microbiota Transplantation With Oral Capsules in Obese Patients. *Clinical Gastroenterology and Hepatology*, doi: 10.1016/j.cgh.2019.07.006.

Allen, A. P. & Smith, A. P. (2015). Chewing gum: cognitive performance, mood, well-being, and associated physiology. *BioMed Research International*, 2015 (654806). doi: 10.1155/2015/654806.

Arumugam, M., Raes, J., Pelletier, E., LePaslier, D., Yamada, T., Mende, D. R., . . . Bork, P. (2011). Enterotypes of the human gut microbiome. *Nature*, 473(7346):274-80. doi: 10.1038/nature09944.

Attaluri, A., Donahoe, R., Valestin, J., Brown, K., & Rao, S. S. (2011). Randomised clinical trial: dried plums (prunes) vs. psyllium for constipation. *Alimentary Pharmacology and Therapeutics*, 33(7):822-8. doi: 10.1111/j.13 652036.2011.04594.x.

Balkwill, F. & Mantovani A. (2001). Inflammation and cancer: back to Virchow? *Lancet*, 357(9255):539-45. doi: 10.1016/S0140-6736(00)04046-0.

Barbara, G., Stanghellini, V., Brandi, G., Cremon, C., Di Nardo, G., De Giorgio, R., & Corinaldesi, R. (2005). Interactions between commensal bacteria and gut sensorimotor function in health and disease. *American Journal of Gastroenterology*, 100(11):2560–2568. doi: 10.1111/j.1572-0241.2005.00230.x.

Basseri, R. J., Basseri, B., Pimentel, M., Chong, K., Youdim, A., Low, K., . . . Mathur, R. (2012). Intestinal methane production in obese individuals is associated with a higher body mass index. *Gastroenterology and Hepatology* 8(1):22-8.

Borody, T., Brandt, L., & Paramsothy, S. (2003). Therapeutic faecal microbiota transplantation: current status and future developments. *Current Opinion in Gastroenterology*, 30(1):97–105. doi: 10.1097/MOG.000000000000002.

Boursi, B., Mamtani, R., Haynes, K., & Yang, Y. (2015). Recurrent antibiotic exposure may promote cancer formation—Another step in understanding the role of the human microbiota? *European Journal of Cancer*, 51(17):2655-64. doi: 10.1016/j.ejca.2015.08.015.

Breban, M., Tap, J., Leboime, A., Said-Nahal, R., Langella, P., Chiocchia, G., Furet J., & Sokol, H. (2017). Faecal microbiota study reveals specific dysbiosis in spondyloarthritis. *Annals of the Rheumatic Diseases*, 76(9):1614-1622. doi: 10.1136/annrheumdis-2016-211064.

Breton, J., Massart, S., Vandamme, P., De Brandt, E., Pot, B., & Foligné, B. (2013). Ecotoxicology inside the gut: impact of heavy metals on the mouse microbiome. *BMC Pharmacol Toxicol*, 14, 62 doi:10.1186/2050-6511-14-62.

Cani, P. & Everard, A. (2015). Talking microbes: When gut bacteria interact with diet and host organs. *Molecular Nutrition & Food Research Review*, 00, 1-9. doi: 10.1002/mnfr.201500406.

Casta-Font, J. & Mas, N. (2016). 'Globesity?' The effects of globalization on obesity and caloric intake. *Food Policy*, (64) 121-132. https://doi.org/10.1016/j.foodpol.2016.10.001

Castex, N., Fioramonti, J., Ducos de Lahitte, J., Luffau, G., More, J., & Bueno, L. (1998). Brain Fos expression and intestinal motor alterations during nematode-induced inflammation in the rat. *American Journal of Physiology*, 274(1 Pt 1):G210-6. PMID: 9458792.

Catassi, C., Alaedini, A., Bojarski, C., Bonaz, B., Bouma, G., Carroccio, A., . . . Sanders, D. (2017). The Overlapping Area of Non-Celiac Gluten Sensitivity

(NCGS) and Wheat-Sensitive Irritable Bowel Syndrome (IBS): An Update. *Nutrients*, 9(11). doi: 10.3390/nu9111268.

Cenit, M., Olivares, M., Codoñer-Franch, P., & Sanz, Y. (2015). Intestinal Microbiota and Celiac Disease: Cause, Consequence or Co-Evolution? *Nutrients*, 7(8): 6900–6923. doi: 10.3390/nu7085314.

Chakŭrski I., Matev, M., Koĭchev, A., Angelova. I., & Stefanov, G. (1981). Treatment of chronic colitis with an herbal combination of *Taraxacum officinale, Hipericum perforatum, Melissa officinaliss, Calendula officinalis* and *Foeniculum vulgare. Vutreshni Bolesti*, 20(6):51-4. PMID: 7336706.

Chassaing, B., Koren, O., Goodrich, J., Poole, A., Srinivasan, S., Ley, R., & Gewirtz, A. T. (2015, 2016). Dietary emulsifiers impact the mouse gut microbiota promoting colitis and metabolic syndrome. *Nature*, 519(7541): 92–96. Correction 2016: 536(7615): 238. doi: 10.1038/nature14232.

Chatterjee, A. & DeVol, R. (2012). Waistlines of the World: The Effect of Information and Communications Technology on Obesity. *Milken Institute Review*, https://assets1b.milkeninstitute.org/assets/Publication/ResearchReport/PDF/Waistlines-of-the-World.pdf.

Chehoud, C., Albenberg, L. G., Judge, C., Hoffmann, C. Grunberg, S., . . .Wu, G. D. (2015). Fungal Signature in the Gut Microbiota of Pediatric Patients with Inflammatory Bowel Disease. *Inflammatory Bowel Diseases*, 21(8):1948-56. doi: 10.1097/.0000000000000454.

Chen, H., Iinuma, M., Onozuka, M. & Kubo, K. Y. (2015). Chewing Maintains Hippocampus-Dependent Cognitive Function. *International Journal of Medical Sciences*, 12(6):502-9. doi: 10.7150/ijms.11911

Chen, H. M., Yu, Y. N., Wang, J. L., Lin, Y. W., Kong, X., Yang, C. Q., . . . Fang, J. Y. (2013). Decreased dietary fiber intake and structural alteration of gut microbiota in patients with advanced colorectal adenoma. *American Journal of Clinical Nutrition*, 97(5):1044-52. doi: 10.MIB3945/ajcn.112.046607.

Cho, I. & Blaser, M. (2012). The human microbiome: at the interface of health and disease. *Nature Reviews, Genetics*, 13(4):260-70. doi: 10.1038/nrg3182

Chocolatewala, N., Chaturvedi, P., & Desale, R. (2010). The role of bacteria in oral cancer. *Indian Journal of Medical and Paediatric Oncology: Official Journal of Indian Society of Medical and Paediatric Oncology*, (4):126-31. doi: 10.4103/0971-5851.76195.

Ciccia, F., Guggino, G., Ferrante, A., Raimondo, S., Bignone, R., Rodolico, V., . . . Giovanni, T. (2016). Interleukin-9 Overexpression and Th9 Polarization Characterize the Inflamed Gut, the Synovial Tissue, and the Peripheral Blood of Patients with Psoriatic Arthritis. *Arthritis & Rheumatology*, doi.org/10.1002/art.39649.

Clegg, M. E., McKenna, P., McClean, C., Davison, G. W., Trinick, T., Duly, E. & Shafat, A. (2011). Gastrointestinal transit, post-prandial lipaemia and satiety following 3 days high-fat diet in men. *European Journal of Clinical Nutrition,* 65(2):240-6. doi: 10.1038/ejcn.2010.235.

Codoñer, F., Ramírez-Bosca, A., Climent, E., Carrión- Gutierrez, M., Guerrero, M., Pérez-Orquín, J., . . . Chenoll, E. (2018). Gut microbial composition in patients with psoriasis. *Scientific Reports,* 8(1):3812. doi: 10.1038/s41598-018-22125-y.

Cohen A., Dreiher, J. & Birkenfeld, S. (2009). Psoriasis associated with ulcerative colitis and Crohn's disease. *Journal of the European Academy of Dermatology and Venereology,* 23, 561–565.10.1111/j.1468-3083.2007.0.

Coit, P. & Sawalha, A. (2016). The human microbiome in rheumatic auto-immune diseases: A comprehensive review. *Clinical Immunology,* 170:70-9. doi: 10.1016/j.clim.2016.07.026.

Collado, C., Donat, E., Ribes-Koninckx, C., Calabuig, M., & Sanz, Y. (2008). Imbalances in faecal and duodenal Bifidobacterium species composition in active and non-active coeliac disease. *BMC Microbiology,* 8:232. doi: 10.1186/1471-2180-8-232.

Collado, M., Calabuig, M., & Sanz, Y. (2007). Differences between the fecal microbiota of coeliac infants and healthy controls. *Current Issues in Intestinal Microbiology*, 8(1):9-14. PMID:17489434.

Collado, M., Donat, E., Ribes-Koninckx, C., Calabuig, M., & Sanz, Y. (2009). Specific duodenal and faecal bacterial groups associated with paediatric coeliac disease. *Journal of Clinical Pathology,* 62(3):264-9. doi: 10.1136/jcp.2008.061366.

Compston, J., Judd, D., Crawley, E., Evans, W., Evans, C., Church, H., Reid, E., & Rhodes J. (1987). Osteoporosis in patients with inflammatory bowel disease. *Gut*, 28(4):410-5. PMCID:PMC1432817.

Costantino, F., Talpin, A., Said-Nahal, R., Goldberg, M., Henny J., Chiocchia, G., & Breban, M. (2015). Prevalence of spondyloarthritis in reference to HLA-B27 in the French population: results of the GAZEL cohort. *Annals of the Rheumatic Diseases,* 74(4):689-93. doi: 10.1136/annrheumdis-2013-204436.

Costello, S., Hughes, P., Waters, O., Bryant, R., Vincent, A., Blatchford, P., . . . Andrews, J. (2019). Effect of Fecal Microbiota Transplantation on 8-Week Remission in Patients with Ulcerative Colitis: A Randomized Clinical Trial. *JAMA,* 15;321(2):156-164. doi: 10.1001/jama.2018.20046.

Coussens, L., Raymond, W., Bergers, G., Laig-Webster, M., Behrendtsen, O., Werb, Z., Caughey, G., & Hanahan, D. (1999). Inflammatory mast cells up-regulate angiogenesis during squamous epithelial carcinogenesis. *Genes & Development,* 13(11):1382-97. PMCID: PMC316772.

Coussens, L. & Werb, Z. (2001). Inflammatory Cells and Cancer: Think Different! *Journal of Experimental Medicine,* 193(6): f23–f26. PMID: 11257144.

Cui, B., Li, P., Xu, L., Zhao, Wang, H., Peng, Z., . . . Zhang, F. (2015). Step-up fecal microbiota transplantation strategy: a pilot study for steroid-dependent ulcerative colitis. *Journal of Translational Medicine,* 13. doi:10.1186/s12967-015-0646-2.

De Filippo, C., Cavalieri, D., Di Paola, M., Ramazzotti, M., Poullet, J.B., Massart, S., . . . Lionetti, P. (2010). Impact of diet in shaping gut microbiota revealed by a comparative study in children from Europe and rural Africa. *Proceedings of the National Academy of Sciences of the United States of America,* 107(33):14691-6. doi: 10.1073/pnas.1005963107.

Di Cagno, R. De Angelis, M., De Pasquale, I., Ndagijimana, M., Vernocchi, P., Ricciuti, P., . . . Francavilla, R. (2011). Duodenal and faecal microbiota of celiac children: molecular, phenotype and metabolome characterization. *BMC Microbiology,* 11: 219. doi: 10.1186/1471-2180-11-219.

Di Cagno, R., Rizzello, C., Gagliardi, F., Ricciuti, P., Ndagijimana, M., Francavilla, R., De Angelis, M. (2009). Different Fecal Microbiotas and Volatile Organic Compounds in Treated and Untreated Children with Celiac Disease. *Applied and Environmental Microbiology,* 5(12): 3963–3971. doi: 10.1128/AEM.02793-08.

Dimidi, E., Christodoulides, S., Fragkos, K. C., Scott, S. M., & Whelan, K. (2014). The effect of probiotics on functional constipation in adults: a systematic review and meta-analysis of randomized controlled trials. *American Journal of Clinical Nutrition,* 100(4):1075-84. doi: 10.3945/ajcn .114.089151.

Dodds, M., Roland, S., Edgar, M., & Thornhill, M. (2015). Saliva: A review of its role in maintaining oral health and preventing dental disease. *Nature: International Journal of Science BDJ Team,* vol. 2, article number: 15123.

Eppinga, H., Konstantinov, S., Peppelenbosch, M., & Thio, H. (2014). The microbiome and psoriatic arthritis. *Current Rheumatology Reports,* 16(3):407. doi: 10.1007/s11926- 013-0407-2.

Fassio, F., Facioni, M. S., & Guagnini, F. (2018) Lactose Maldigestion, Malabsorption, and Intolerance: A Comprehensive Review with a Focus on Current Management and Future Perspectives. *Nutrients,* 10(11). doi: 10.3390/nu10111599.

Finegold, S., Summanen, P., Downes. J., Corbett, K., & Komoriya, T. (2017). Detection of Clostridium perfringens toxin genes in the gut microbiota of autistic children. *Anaerobe,* 45:133-137. doi: 10.1016/j.anaerobe.2017.02.008.

Flint, H., Scott, K., Louis, P., & Duncan, S. (2012). The Nature Reviews, *Gastroenterology & Hepatology* 9(10):577-89. doi: 10.1038/nrgastro.2012 .156.

Forootan, M., Bagheri, N., & Darvishi, M. (2018). Chronic constipation: A review of literature., *Medicine,* (Baltimore) 2018 May; 97(20): e10631. doi: 10.1097/MD.0000000000010631.

Frank, D. N., Robertson, C. E., Hamm, C. M., Kpadeh, Z., Zhang, T., Chen, H., Li, E. (2011). Disease phenotype and genotype are associated with shifts in intestinal-associated microbiota in inflammatory bowel diseases. *Inflammatory Bowel Disease,* 17(1): 10.1002/ibd.21339. doi: 10.1002/ ibd.21339.

Furuya-Kanamori, L., McKenzie, S., Yakob, L., Clark, J., Paterson, D., Riley, T., & Clements, A. (2015). Clostridium difficile Infection Seasonality: Patterns across Hemispheres and Continents—A Systematic Review. *PLoS One,* 0(3). doi: 10.1371/journal.pone.0120730.

Gao, Z., Tseng, C., Strober, B., Pei, Z. & Blaser, M. (2008). Substantial Alterations of the Cutaneous Bacterial Biota in Psoriatic Lesions. *PlusOne*, https://doi.org/10.1371/journal.pone.0002719.

Garborg, K., Waagsbø, B., Stallemo, A., Matre, J., & Sundøy, A. (2010). Results of faecal donor instillation therapy for recurrent Clostridium difficile-associated diarrhoea. *Scandinavian Journal of Infectious Diseases*, 42(11-12):857-61. doi: 10.3109/00365548.2010.499541.

Gerritsen, J., Smidt, H., Rijkers, G. T., & de Vos, W. M. (2011). Intestinal microbiota in human health and disease: the impact of probiotics. *Genes and Nutrition*, 6(3):209-40. doi: 10.1007/s12263-011-0229-7.

Goehler, L., Park, S., Opitz, N., Lyte, M., & Gaykema, R. (2007). Campylobacter jejuni infection increases anxiety- like behavior in the holeboard: possible anatomical substrates for viscerosensory modulation of exploratory behavior. *Brain, Behavior & Immunity*, 22(3):354-66. doi: 10.1016/j.bbi.2007.08.009.

Goodrich, J., Davenport, E., Clark, A., & Ley, R. (2017). The relationship between the human genome and microbiome comes into view. *Annual Review of Genetics*, 51. doi: 10.1146/annurev-genet-110711-155532.

Gopalakrishnan, V., Spencer, C., Nezi, L., Reuben, A., Andrews, M., Karpinets, T., . . . Wargo, J. (2018). *Science*, 359(6371):97-103. doi: 10.1126/science. aan4236.

Gustafsson, A., Berstad, A., Lund-Tønnesen, S., Midtvedt, T., & Norin, E. (1999). The effect of faecal enema on five microflora-associated characteristics in patients with antibiotic-associated diarrhoea. *Scandinavian Journal of Gasteroenterology*, 34(6):580-6. PMID:10440607.

Hamilton, M., Weingarden, A., Sadowsky, M., & Khoruts, A. (2012). Standardized frozen preparation for transplantation of fecal microbiota for recurrent *Clostridium difficile* infection. *American Journal of Gastroenterology*, 107(5):761-7. doi: 10.1038/ajg.2011.482.

Hammond, E. & Donker, E. (2013). Antibacterial effect of Manuka honey on Clostridium difficile. *BMC Research Notes*, 6:188. doi. org/10.1186/1756-0500-6-188.

Hayden, M. & Ghosh S. (2008). Shared principles in NF-kappaB signaling. *Cell*, 132(3):344-62. doi: 10.1016/j.cell.2008.01.020.

Ho, K. S., Tan, C.Y., Mohd Daud, M.A., & Seow-Choen, F. (2012). Stopping or reducing dietary fiber intake reduces constipation and its associated symptoms, *Journal of Gastroenterology*, 18(33):4593-6. doi: 10.3748/wjg. v18.i33.4593.

Hoffman, M., Butler, T., & Shaver, T. (1998). Colonoscopy without sedation. *Journal of Clinical Gastroenterology*, 26(4):279-82. PMID:9649011.

Hsu A., Aronoff, D. M., Phipps, J., Goel, D., & Mancuso, P. (2018). Leptin improves pulmonary bacterial clearance and survival in ob/ob mice during pneumococcal pneumonia. *Clinical and Experimental Immunology*, 150(2). doi: 10.1111/j.1365-2249.2007.03491.x.

Jiang, W., Wu, N., Wang, X., Chi, Y., Zhang, Y., Qiu, X., . . . Liu, Y. (2015). Dysbiosis gut microbiota associated with inflammation and impaired mucosal immune function in intestine of humans with non-alcoholic fatty liver disease. *Scientific Reports*, 5:8096. doi: 10.1038/srep08096.

Kang, D., Adams, J., Coleman, D., Pollard, E., Maldonado, J., McDonough-Means, S., Caporaso, J. G., & Krajmalnik-Brown, R. (2019). Long-term benefit of Microbiota Transfer Therapy on autism symptoms and gut microbiota. *Scientific Reports*, 9: 5821. doi: 10.1038/s41598-019-42183-0.

Kang, D., EsraIlhan, Z., Isern, N., Hoyt, D., Howsmon, D., Shaffer, M., Krajmalnik-Brown, R. (2017). Differences in fecal microbial metabolites and microbiota of children with autism spectrum disorders. *Anaerobe*, (49)121-131. https://doi.org/10.1016/j.anaerobe.2017.12.007.

Kao, D., Roach, B., Silva, M., Beck, P., Rioux, K., & Louie T. (2017). Effect of Oral Capsule- vs Colonoscopy-Delivered Fecal Microbiota Transplantation on Recurrent Clostridium difficile Infection: A Randomized Clinical Trial. *JAMA*, 318(20):1985-1993. doi:10.1001/jama.2017.17077.

Karlsson, F., Fåk, F., Nookaew, I., Tremaroli, V., Fagerberg, B., Petranovic, D., Bäckhed. F., & Nielsen, J. (2012). Symptomatic atherosclerosis is associated with an altered gut metagenome. *Nature Communications*, 3 (1245). doi: 10.1038/ncomms2266.

Kelly, P. (2018). A new immune syndrome identified. *Science,* 362 (6416):789-790. doi: 10.1126/science.362.6416.789-b.

Khalif, I. L., Quigley, E. M., Konovitch, E. A., & Maximova, I. D. (2005). Alterations in the colonic flora and intestinal permeability and evidence of immune activation in chronic constipation. *Digestive and Liver Disease: official journal of the Italian society of gastroenterology and the Italian association for the study of the liver*, 37(11):838-49. doi:10.1016/j.dld.2005.06.008.

Khan, R., Lawson, A.D., Minnich, L.L., Martin, K., Nasir, A., Emmett, M.K., Welch, C.A., & Udall, J.N. Jr. (2009). Gastrointestinal norovirus infection associated with exacerbation of inflammatory bowel disease. *Journal of Pediatric Gastroenterology and Nutrition*, 48(3):328-33. doi:10.1097/mpg.0b013e31818255cc.

Kim, S.M. (2016). Human papilloma virus in oral cancer. *Journal of the Korean Association of Oral Maxillofacial Surgeons*, 42(6):327-336. doi: 10.5125/jkaoms.2016.42.6.327.

Kirgizov, I. V., Sukhorukov, A. M., Dudarev, V. A., & Istomin, A. A. (2001). Hemostasis in children with dysbacteriosis in chronic constipation. *Clinical and Applied Thrombosis/Hemostasis*, 7(4):335-8. PMID:11697720.

Klement, E., Cohen, R., Boxman, J., Joseph, A., & Reif, S. (2004). Breastfeeding and risk of inflammatory bowel disease: a systematic review with meta-analysis. *American Journal of Clinical Nutrition*, 80(5):1342-52. doi: 10.1093/ajcn/80.5.1342.

Knights, D., Parfrey, L., Zaneveld, J., Lozupone, C., & Knight, R. (2011). Human-associated microbial signatures: examining their predictive value. *Cell Host & Microbe*, 10(4):292-6. doi: 10.1016/j.chom.2011.09.003.

Kragsnaes, M., Kjeldsen, J., Horn, H., Munk, H., Pedersen, F., Holt, H., . . . Ellingsen, T. (2017). Efficacy and safety of faecal microbiota transplantation in patients with psoriatic arthritis: protocol for a 6-month, double-blind, randomised, placebo-controlled trial. *BMJ Open*, 8(4). doi: 10.1136/bmjopen-2017-019231.

Kuenstner, J.T., Naser, S., Chamberlin, W., Borody, T., Graham, D. Y., McNees, A., . . . Kuenstner, L. (2017). The Consensus from the Mycobacterium avium spp. Paratuberculosis (MAP) Conference 2017. *Frontiers in Public Health*, 5 (208). doi: 10.3389/fpubh.2017.00208.

Kugeler, K., Griffith, K., Gould, L., Kochanek, K., Delorey, M., Biggerstaff, B., & Mead, P. (2011). A review of death certificates listing Lyme disease as a cause of death in the United States. *Clinical Infectious Diseases*, 52(3):364-7. doi: 10.1093/cid/ciq157.

Kuper, H., Adami, H., & Trichopoulos, D. (2000). Infections as a major preventable cause of human cancer. *Journal of Internal Medicine*, 248(3):171-83. PMID:10971784.

Lach, G., Schellekens, H., Dinan, T., & Cryan, J. (2018). Anxiety, Depression, and the Microbiome: A Role for Gut Peptides. *Neurotherapeutics*, 15(1):36-59. doi: 10.1007/s13311-017-0585-0.

Lam, V., Su, J., Koprowski, S., Hsu, A., Tweddell, J., . . . Baker, J. (2012). Intestinal microbiota determine severity of myocardial infarction in rats. *Federation of American Societies for Experimental Biology*, 26(4). doi: 10.1096/fj.11-197921.

Le Chatelier, E., Nielsen, T., Qin, J., Prifti, E., Hildebrand, F., Falony, G., . . . Pedersen, O. (2013) Richness of human gut microbiome correlates with metabolic markers. *Nature*, 500(7464):541-6. doi: 10.1038/nature12506.

Ley, R., Bäckhed, F., Turnbaugh, P., Lozupone, C., Knight, R., & Gordon J.(2005). Obesity alters gut microbial ecology. *Proceedings of the National Academy of Sciences of the USA*, 102(31):11070. doi: 10.1016/j.cell.2018.10.029.

Li, J., Chassaing, B., Malik, A., Vaccaro, C., Luo, T., Adams, J., . . . Pacifici, R. (2016). Sex steroid deficiency–associated bone loss is microbiota dependent and prevented by probiotics. *The Journal of Clinical Investigation*, 126(6):2049–2063. https://doi.org/10.1172/JCI86062.

Liguori, G., Lamas, B., Richard, M., Brandi, G., da Costa, G., Hoffmann, T., . . . Sokol, H. (2016). Fungal Dysbiosis in Mucosa-associated Microbiota of Crohn's Disease Patients. *Journal of Crohn's and Colitis*, 10(3):296-305. doi: 10.1093/ecco-jcc/jjv209.

Limon, J. J., Tang, J., Dalin, L., & Underhill, D. M. (2019). Malassezia Is Associated with Crohn's Disease and Exacerbates Colitis in Mouse Models. *Cell, Host & Microbe*, 25(3). doi: 10.1016/j.chom.2019.01.007.

Lloyd-Price, J., Abu-Ali, G., & Huttenhower, C. (2016). The healthy human microbiome. *Genome Medicine*, 8(51). doi.org/10.1186/s13073-016-0307-y.

Lochhead, R., Strle, K., Kim, N., Kohler, M., Arvikar, S., Aversa, J., & Steere, A. (2017). MicroRNA expression shows inflammatory dysregulation and tumor-like proliferative responses in joints of patients with post-infectious Lyme arthritis. *Arthritis & Rheumatology*, 69(5): 1100–1110. doi: 10.1002/art.40039.

Lyte, M., Li, W., Opitz, N., Gaykema, R., & Goehler, L. (2006) Induction of anxiety-like behavior in mice during the initial stages of infection with the agent of murine colonic hyperplasia *Citrobacter rodentium*. *Physiology & Behavior,* 89(3):350-7. doi: 10.1016/j.physbeh.2006.06.019.

Lyte, M., Varcoe, J., & Bailey M. (1998). Anxiogenic effect of subclinical bacterial infection in mice in the absence of overt immune activation. *Physiology & Behavior,* 65(1):63-8. PMID: 9811366.

Mancuso, P., Gottschalk, A., Phare, S., Peters-Golden, M., Lukacs, N., & Huffnagle, G. (2002). Leptin-deficient mice exhibit impaired host defense in gram-negative pneumonia. *Journal of Immunology,* 168(8):4018-24. PMID:11937559.

Manichanh, C., Eck, A., Varela, E., Roca, J., Clemente, J. C., González, A., Knights, D., . . . Azpiroz, F. (2014). Anal gas evacuation and colonic microbiota in patients with flatulence: effect of diet. *Gut,* 63(3):401-8. doi: 10.1136/gutjnl-2012-303013.

Matson, V., Fessler, J., Bao, R., Chongsuwat, T., Zha, Y., Alegre, M., Luke, J., & Gajewski, T. (2018). The commensal microbiome is associated with anti-PD-1 efficacy in metastatic melanoma patients. *Science,* 359(6371):104-108. doi: 10.1126/science.aao3290.

Menni, C., Jackson, M., Pallister, T., Steves, C., Spector, T., & Valdes, A. (2017). Gut microbiome diversity and high- fibre intake are related to lower long-term weight gain. *International Journal of Obesity,* 41(7):1099-1105. doi: 10.1038/ijo.2017.66.

Merve, H., Sevilay, K., Sibel, O., Başak, B., Ceren, C., Demirci, T., & Cüneyt, A. (2017). Psoriasis and Genetics. *Intechopen,* intechopen.com/books/an-interdisciplinary-approach-to-psoriasis/psoriasis-and-genetics. doi: 10.5772/intechopen.68344.

Meylan, E., Tschopp, J., & Karin, M. (2006). Intracellular pattern recognition receptors in the host response. *Nature,* 442(7098):39-44.

Moayyedi, P., Marshall, J., Yuan, Y., & Hunt, R. (2014). Canadian Association of Gastroenterology position statement: Fecal microbiota transplant therapy. *Canadian Journal of Gastroenterology and Hepatology,* 28(2). PMCID: PMC4071888.

Moeller, A. Li, Y., Mpoudi Ngole, E., Ahuka-Mundeke, S., Lonsdorf, E., Pusey, A., Peeters, M., Hahn, B., & Ochman, H. (2014). Rapid changes in the gut microbiome during human evolution. *Proceedings of the National Academy of Sciences of the United States of America,* 111(46):16431-5. doi: 10.1073/pnas.1419136111.

Morgan, X., Tickle, T., Sokol, H., Gevers, D., Devaney, K. L., . . . Huttenhower, C. (2012). Dysfunction of the intestinal microbiome in inflammatory bowel disease and treatment. *Genome Biology,* 13(9):R79. doi: 10.1186/gb-2012-13-9-r79.

Moshyedi, K., Josephs, M., Abdalla, E., Mackay, S., Edwards, C., Copeland, E., & Moldawer, L. (1998). Increased leptin expression in mice with bacterial peritonitis is partially regulated by tumor necrosis factor alpha. *Infection and Immunity,* 166(4):1800-2. PMCID:PMC108125.

Nakano K., Nomura, R., Matsumoto, M., & Ooshima, T. (2010). Roles of oral bacteria in cardiovascular diseases—from molecular mechanisms to clinical cases: Cell-surface structures of novel serotype k *Streptococcus mutans* strains and their correlation to virulence. *Journal of Pharmacological Sciences,* 113:120-125.

Nehra, A. , Alexander, J., Loftus, C., & Nehra, V. (2018}. Proton Pump Inhibitors: Review of Emerging Concerns. *Mayo Clinic Proceedings,* 93(2):240-246. doi: 10.1016/j.mayocp.2017.10.022.

Ng, Siew C. (2016). Emerging Trends of Inflammatory Bowel Disease in Asia. *Gastroenterol Hepatology (N Y),* 12(3): 193–196. PMID: 27231449.

Noach, L., Rolf, T., & Tytgat, G. (1994). Electron microscopic study of association between *Helicobacter pylori* and gastric and duodenal mucosa. *Journal of Clinical Pathology,* 47(8): 699–704. PMID: 7962619.

Ohara, T. & Suzutani, T. (2018). Efficacy of fecal microbiota transplantation in a patient with chronic intractable constipation. *Clinical Case Reports,* 6(11):2029-2032. doi: 10.1002/ccr3.1798.

Pachner, A. & Steiner, I. (2007). Lyme neuroborreliosis: infection, immunity, and inflammation. *The Lancet Neurology,* doi:10.1016/S1474-4422(07)70128 -X.

Paramsothy, S., Nielsen, S., Kamm, M., Deshpande, N.P., Faith, J.J., . . . Kaakoush, N. O., (2019). Specific Bacteria and Metabolites Associated With

Response to Fecal Microbiota Transplantation in Patients With Ulcerative Colitis. *Gastroenterology*, 156(5):1440-1454. https://doi.org/10.1053/j.gastro.2018.12.001.

Paramsothy, S., Borody, T., Lin, E., Finlayson, S., Walsh, A. J., Samuel, D., ... Kamm, M. (2015). Donor Recruitment for Fecal Microbiota Transplantation. *Inflammatory Bowel Disease*, 21(7).https://academic,oup.com/ibdjournal/article- abstract/21/7/1600/4604260.

Paramsothy, S., Paramsothy, R., Rubin, D., Kamm, M., Kaakoush, N., Mitchell, H. & Castaño-Rodríguez, N. (2017). Faecal Microbiota Transplantation for Inflammatory Bowel Disease: A Systematic Review and Meta-analysis. *Journal of Crohn's and Colitis*, 11(10):1180-1199. doi: 10.1093/ecco-jcc/jjx063.

Parnell, J. & Reimer, R. (2009). Weight loss during oligofructose supplementation is associated with decreased ghrelin and increased peptide YY in overweight and obese adults. *American Journal of Clinical Nutrition*, 89(6):1751-9. doi: 10.3945/ajcn.2009.27465.

Pei, Z., Yang, L., Peek, Jr., R., Levine, S., Pride, D., & Blaser, M. (2005). Bacterial biota in reflux esophagitis and Barrett's esophagus. *World Journal of Gastroenterology*, 11(46): 7277–7283. doi: 10.3748/wjg.v11.i46.7277.

Perez-Muñoz, M., Arrieta, M., Ramer-Tait, A. & Walter, J. (2017). A critical assessment of the "sterile womb" and "in utero colonization" hypotheses: implications for research on the pioneer infant microbiome. *Microbiome*, 5(1). doi: 10.1186/s40168-017-0268-4.

Plottel, C., & Blaser, M. (2011). Microbiome and malignancy. *Cell Host & Microbe*, 10(4):324-35. doi: 10.1016/j.chom.2011.10.003.

Pushalkar, S., Hundeyin, M., Daley, D., Zambirinis, C.P., Kurz, E., Mishra ... Miller, G. (2018). The Pancreatic Cancer Microbiome Promotes Oncogenesis by Induction of Innate and Adaptive Immune Suppression. *Cancer Discovery*, DOI: 10.1158/2159-8290.CD-17-1134.

Queipo-Ortuño, M., Seoane, L., Murri, M., Pardo, M., Gomez-Zumaquero, J., Cardona, F., Casanueva, F., & Tinahones, F. (2013). Gut microbiota composition in male rat models under different nutritional status and physical activity and its association with serum leptin and ghrelin levels. *PLoS One*, 8(5). doi: 10.1371/journal.pone.0065465.

Rajala, M., Patterson, C., Opp, J., Foltin, S. , Young, V., & Myers M. (2014). Leptin acts independently of food intake to modulate gut microbial composition in male mice. *Endocrinology*, 155(3):748-57. doi: 10.1210/ en.2013-1085.

Ramai, D., Zakhia, K., Ofosu, A., Ofori, E., & Reddy, M. (2019). Fecal microbiota transplantation: donor relation, fresh or frozen, delivery methods, cost-effectiveness. *Annals of Gasteroenterology*, 32(1):30-38. doi: 10.20524/ aog.2018.0328.

Remely, M., Hippe, B., Geretschlaeger, I., Stegmayer. S., Hoefinger, I., & Haslberger, A. (2015). Increased gut microbiota diversity and abundance of *Faecalibacterium prausnitzii* and *Akkermansia* after fasting: a pilot study. *Wiener Klinische Wochenschrift*, 127(9-10):394-8. doi: 10.1007/ s00508-015-0755-1.

Revaiah, P. C., Kochhar, R., Rana, S. V., Berry, N., Ashat, M., Dhaka, N., Rami Reddy, Y., & Sinha, S. K. (2018). Risk of small intestinal bacterial overgrowth in patients receiving proton pump inhibitors versus proton pump inhibitors plus prokinetics. *Journal of Gastroenterology and Hepatology*, 2(2):47-53. doi: 10.1002/jgh3.12045.

Rojas, D., Smith, J., Benkers, T. , Camou, S., Reite. M., Rogers, S. (2004). Hippocampus and amygdala volumes in parents of children with autistic disorder. *American Journal of Psychiatry*, 161(11):2038-44. doi:10.1176/ appi.ajp.161.11.2038.

Rossen, N., Fuentes, S., van der Spek, M., Tijssen, J., Hartman, J., Duflou, A., . . . Ponsioen, C. (2015). Findings from a Randomized Controlled Trial of Fecal Transplantation for Patients with Ulcerative Colitis. *Gastroenterology*, 149(1):110-118.e4. doi: 10.1053/j.gastro.2015.03.045.

Routy, B., Le Chatelier, E., Derosa, L., Duong, C., Alou, M., Daillère, R., . . . Zitvogel, L. (2018). Gut microbiome influences efficacy of PD-1-based immunotherapy against epithelial tumors. *Science*, 359(6371):91-97. doi: 10.1126/science.aan3706.

Sanz, Y. (2015). Microbiome and Gluten. *Annals of Nutrition and Metabolism*, 28-41. doi: 10.1159/000440991.

Sapone, A., Bai, J. C., Ciacci, C., Dolinsek, J., Green, P. H., Hadjivassiliou, M., . . . Fasano, A. (2012). Spectrum of gluten-related disorders:

consensus on new nomenclature and classification. *BMC Medicine*, 10(13). doi: 10.1186/1741-7015-10-13.

Sarraf, P., Frederich, R., Turner, E., Ma, G., Jaskowiak, N., Rivet, D., . . . Alexander, H. (1997). Multiple cytokines and acute inflammation raise mouse leptin levels: potential role in inflammatory anorexia. *Journal of Experimental Medicine*, 185(1):171-5. PMCID:PMC2196098.

Sartor, R. (2014). The intestinal microbiota in inflammatory bowel diseases. *Nestle Nutritional Workshop Series*, 79:29-39. doi: 10.1159/000360674.

Sartor, R. & Wu, G. (2017). Roles for Intestinal Bacteria, Viruses, and Fungi in Pathogenesis of Inflammatory Bowel Diseases and Therapeutic Approaches. *Gastroenterology*, 152(2):327-339.e4. doi: 10.1053/j.gastro.2016.10.012.

Sato, W., Kochiyama, T., Uono, S., Yoshimura, S., Kubota, Y., Sawada, R., Sakihama, M. & Toichi, M. (2017). Reduced Gray Matter Volume in the Social Brain Network in Adults with Autism Spectrum Disorder. *Frontiers in Human Neuroscience*, 11:395. doi: 10.3389/fnhum.2017.00395.

Scheiman J., Luber, J.M., Chavkin, T.A., MacDonald, T., . . . Kostic, A.D. (2019). Meta-omics analysis of elite athletes identifies a performance-enhancing microbe that functions via lactate metabolism. *Nature Medicine*, 25(7):1104-1109. doi: 10.1038/s41591-019-0485-4.

Scher, J., Sczesnak, A., Longman, R., Segata, N., Ubeda, C., Bielski, C., . . . Littman, D. (2013). Expansion of intestinal Prevotella copri correlates with enhanced susceptibility to arthritis. *eLife,* doi:10.7554/eLife.01202/.

Scher, J., Ubeda, C., Artacho, A., Attur, M., Isaac, S., Reddy, S., . . . Abramson, S. (2015). Decreased bacterial diversity characterizes the altered gut microbiota in patients with psoriatic arthritis, resembling dysbiosis in inflammatory bowel disease. *Arthritis & Rheumatology*, (1):128-39. doi: 10.1002/art.38892.

Schippa, S., Iebba, V., Barbato, M., Di Nardo, G., Totino, V., Checchi, M., . . . Conte, M. (2010). A distinctive 'microbial signature' in celiac pediatric patients. *BMC Microbiology*, 10:175. doi: 10.1186/1471-2180-10-175.

Segal, L. & Blaser, M. (2014). A Brave New World: The Lung Microbiota in an Era of Change. *Annals of the American Thoracic Society*, 11(Suppl 1): S21–S27. doi: 10.1513/AnnalsATS.201306-189MG.

Siegel, R., Naishadham, D. & Jemal, A. (2012). Cancer statistics. *CA: A Cancer Journal for Clinicians*, 62: 10–29. doi: 10.3322/caac.20138.

Sjögren, K., Engdahl, C., Henning, P., Lerner, U. , Tremaroli, V., Lagerquist, M., Bäckhed, F., & Ohlsson C. (2012). The gut microbiota regulates bone mass in mice. *Journal of Bone and Mineral Research*, 27(6):1357-67. doi: 10.1002/jbmr.1588.

Smeekens, S., Huttenhower, C., Riza, A., van de Veerdonk, F., Zeeuwen, P., Schalkwijk, J.,... Gevers, D. (2014). Skin microbiome imbalance in patients with STAT1/STAT3 defects impairs innate host defense responses. *Journal of Innate Immunity*, 6(3):253-62. doi: 10.1159/000351912.

Sokol, H., Leducq, V., Aschard, H., Pham, H., Jegou, S., Landman, C.,... Cohen, D. (2017) *Fungal microbiota dysbiosis in IBD. Gut*, 66:1039-1048. http://dx.doi.org/10.1136/gutjnl-2015-310746.

Soloski, M., Crowder, L., Lahey, L., Wagner, C., Robinson, W., & Aucott, J. (2014). Serum inflammatory mediators as markers of human Lyme disease activity. *PLoS One*, 9(4):e93243. doi: 10.1371/journal.pone.0093243.

Sonoyama, K., Fujiwara, R., Takemura, N., Ogasawara, T., Watanabe, J., Ito, H., & Morita, T. (2009). Response of gut microbiota to fasting and hibernation in Syrian hamsters. *Applied and Environmental Microbiology*, 75(20):6451-6. doi: 10.1128/AEM.00692-09.

Soon, I., Molodecky, N., Rabi, D., Ghali, W., Barkema, H., & Kaplan, G. (2012). The relationship between urban environment and the inflammatory bowel diseases: a systematic review and meta-analysis. *BMC Gastroenterology*, 12(51). doi: 10.1186/1471-230X-12-51.

Spinler, J. K., Brown, A., Ross, C. L., Boonma, P., Connor, M., & Savidge T.C. (2016). Administration of Probiotic Kefir to Mice with *Clostridium difficile* Infection Exacerbates Disease. *Anaerobe*, 40: 54–57. doi: 10.1016/j.anaerobe.2016.05.008.

Staley, C., Vaughn, B., Graiziger, C., Singroy, S., Hamilton, M., Yao, D.,... Sadowsky, M. (2017). Community dynamics drive punctuated engraftment of the fecal microbiome following transplantation using freeze-dried, encapsulated fecal microbiota. *Gut Microbes*, 8(3):276-288. doi: 10.1080/19490976.2017.1299310.

Starkey, J., MacPherson, J., Bolgiano, D., Simon, E., Zuck, T., & Sayers, M. (1989). Markers for transfusion-transmitted disease in different groups of blood donors. *JAMA*, 1989 Dec 22-29;262(24):3452-4. PMID: 2585691.

Sun, L., Ma, L., Ma, Y., Zhang, F., Zhao, C., & Nie, Y. (2018). Insights into the role of gut microbiota in obesity: pathogenesis, mechanisms, and therapeutic perspectives. *Protein Cell*, 9(5): 397–403. doi: 10.1007/s13238-018-0546-3.

Takagi, T., Naito, Y., Inoue, R., Kashiwagi, S., Uchiyama, K., Mizushima. K., . . . Itoh, Y. (2018). The influence of long-term use of proton pump inhibitors on the gut microbiota: an age-sex-matched case-control study. *Journal of Clinical Biochemistry and Nutrition*, 62(1):100-105. doi: 10.3164/jcbn.17-78.

Tan, J., McKenzie, C., Potamitis, M., Thorburn, A. N., Mackay, C. R., & Macia, L. (2014) The role of short-chain fatty acids in health and disease. *Advances in Immunology*, 121:91–119. doi: 10.1016/B978-0-12- 800100-4.00003-9.

Tang, W., Wang, Z., Kennedy, D., Wu, Y., Buffa, J., Agatisa- Boyle, B., . . . Hazen, S. (2015). Gut microbiota-dependent trimethylamine N-oxide (TMAO) pathway contributes to both development of renal insufficiency and mortality risk in chronic kidney disease. *Circulation Research*, 116(3):448-55. doi: 10.1161/CIRCRESAHA.116.305360.

Terveer, E., van Beurden, Y., Goorhuis, A., Seegers, J., Bauer, M., van Nood, E., . . . Kuijper, E. (2017). How to: Establish and run a stool bank. *Clinical Microbiology and Infection*, 924-930. doi: 10.1016/j.cmi.2017.05.015.

Tett, A., Pasolli, E., Farina, S., Truong, D., Asnicar, F., Zolfo, M., . . . Segata, N. (2017). Unexplored diversity and strain-level structure of the skin microbiome associated with psoriasis. *NPJ Biofilms Microbiomes*, 3:14. doi: 10.1038/s41522-017-0022-5.

Turnbaugh, J., Bäckhed, F., Fulton, L., & Gordon, J. (2008). Diet-induced obesity is linked to marked but reversible alterations in the mouse distal gut microbiome. *Cell Host & Microbe*, 3(4):213-23. doi: 10.1016/j.chom.2008.02.015.

Valles-Colomer, M., Falony, G., Darzi, Y., Tigchelaar, E., Wang, J., Tito, R., . . . Raes, J. (2019). The Neuroactive Potential of the Human Gut Microbiota in Quality of Life and Depression. *Nature Microbiology*, 4(4):623-632. doi: 10.1038/s41564-018-0337-x.

Vangay, P., Johnson, A., Ward, T., Al-Ghalith, G., Shields-Cutler, R., Hillmann, B., & Knights D. (2018). *Cell*, 175(4):962-972. doi: 10.1016/j.cell.2018.10.029.

Venkova, T., Yeo, C.C., & Espinosa, M. (2018). Editorial: The Good, The Bad, and The Ugly: Multiple Roles of Bacteria in Human Life. *Frontiers in Microbiology*, 9(1702). doi: 10.3389/fmicb.2018.01702.

Volta, U., Caio, G., Tovoli, F., & De Giorgio, R. (2013). Non- celiac gluten sensitivity: questions still to be answered despite increasing awareness. *Cellular and Molecular Immunology*, 10(5):383-92. doi: 10.1038/cmi.2013.28.

Vrieze, A., Van Nood, E., Holleman, F., Salojärvi, J., Kootte, R., Bartelsman, J., . . . Nieuwdorp, M. (2012). *Gastroenterology*, 143(4):913-6. doi: 10.1053/j.gastro.2012.06.031.

Waller, P., Gopal, P., Leyer, G., Ouwehand, A., Reifer, C., Stewart, M., & Miller, L. (2011). Dose-response effect of *Bifidobacterium lactis* HN019 on whole gut transit time and functional gastrointestinal symptoms in adults. *Scandinavian Journal of Gastroenterology*, 46(9):1057-64. doi: 10.3109/00365521.2011.584895.

Wassenaar, T. & Zimmermann, K. (2018). Lipopolysaccharides in Food, Food Supplements, and Probiotics: Should We be Worried? *European Journal of Microbiology and Immunology*, 8(3):63-69. doi: 10.1556/1886.2018.00017.

Wu, R., Pasyk, M., Wang, B., Forsythe, P., Bienenstock, J., Mao, Y., Sharma, P., Stanisz, A. & Kunze, W. (2013). Spatiotemporal maps reveal regional differences in the effects on gut motility for *Lactobacillus reuteri* and *rhamnosus* strains. *Neurogastroenterology and Motility: the official journal of the European gastrointestinal motility society*, 25(3):e205-14. doi: 10.1111/nmo.12072.

Yagi, T., Ueda, H., Amitani, H., Asakawa, A., Miyawaki, S., & Inui, A. (2012). The role of ghrelin, salivary secretions, and dental care in eating disorders. *Nutrients*, 4(8):967- 89.

Yang, F., Ning, K., Chang, X., Yuan, X., Tu, Q., Yuan, T., Deng, Y., . . . Xu, J. (2014). Saliva Microbiota Carry Caries- Specific Functional Gene Signatures. *PLoS One*, 9(2). doi: 10.1371/journal.pone.0076458

Yang, T., Santisteban, M., Rodriguez, V., Li, E., Ahmari, N., Carvajal, J., . . . Mohamadzadeh, M. (2015). Gut dysbiosis is linked to hypertension. *Hypertension*, 65(6):1331-40. doi: 10.1161/HYPERTENSIONAHA.115.05315.

Yatsunenko, T., Rey, F., Manary, M., Trehan, I., Dominguez- Bello, M., Contreras, M., . . . J. (2012). Human gut microbiome viewed across age and geography. *Nature,* 9;486(7402):222-7. doi: 10.1038/nature11053.

Zackular, J., Baxter, N., Iverson, K., Sadler, W., Petrosino, J., Chen, G., & Schloss, P. (2013). The gut microbiome modulates colon tumorigenesis. *MBio,* 4(6). doi: 10.1128/mBio.00692-13.

Zhao, S., Liu, W., Wang, J., Shi, J., Sun, Y., Wang, W., . . . Jie, H. (2016). *Akkermansia muciniphila* improves metabolic profiles by reducing inflammation in chow diet-fed mice. *Journal of Molecular Endocrinology,* 58(1). doi: 10.1530/JME-16-0054.

Zhou, Y., Chen, H., He, H., Du, Y., Hu, J., Li, Y., . . . Nie, Y. (2016) Increased *Enterococcus faecalis* infection is associated with clinically active Crohn disease. *Medicine,* (95)39. doi: 10.1097/MD.0000000000005019.

Zhu, Q., Jin, Z., Wu, W., Gao, R., Guo, B., Gao, Z., . . . Qin, H. (2014). Analysis of the intestinal lumen microbiota in an animal model of colorectal cancer. *PLoS One,* 9(6):e90849. doi: 10.1371/journal.pone.0090849.

Zhu, Y. & Hollis, J. H. (2014). Increasing the number of chews before swallowing reduces meal size in normal-weight, overweight, and obese adults. *Journal of the Academy of Nutrition and Dietetics,* 114(6):926-31. doi: 10.1016/j.jand.2013.08.020.

Zipursky, J., Sidorsky, T., Freedman, C., Sidorsky, M., & Kirkland, K. (2012). Patient attitudes toward the use of fecal microbiota transplantation in the treatment of recurrent *Clostridium difficile infection. Clinical Infectious Diseases,* 55(12):1652-8. doi: 10.1093/cid/cis809.

Zoppi, G., Cinquetti, M., Luciano, A., Benini, A., Muner, A., & Bertazzoni, M. (1998). The intestinal ecosystem in chronic functional constipation. *Acta Paediatrica,* 87(8):836-41. PMID: 9736230.

INDEX